Prevention and Health: Directions for Policy and Practice

Prevention and Health: Directions for Policy and Practice

Alfred H. Katz
Jared A. Hermalin
Robert E. Hess
Editors

The Haworth Press
New York • London

Prevention and Health: Directions for Policy and Practice, has also been published as *Prevention in Human Services*, Volume 5, Number 1, Fall/Winter 1986.

The Haworth Press, Inc., 12 West '32 Street, New York, NY 10001
EUROSPAN/Haworth, 3 Henrietta Street, London WC2E 8LU England

Library of Congress Cataloging-in-Publication Data

Prevention and health.

   "Has also been published as Prevention in human services, volume 5, number 1, fall/winter 1986"—T.p. verso.
   Includes bibliographies.
   1. Medicine, Prevention—Case studies. I. Katz, Alfred H. (Alfred Hyman), 1916–   . II. Hermalin, Jared. III. Hess, Robert, 1948–   . [DNLM: 1. Health Policy. 2. Preventive Health Services. 3. Primary Prevention. W1 PR497 v.5 no. 1/WA 108 P9415]
RA427.P74   1987   614.4'4   87-17634
ISBN 0-86656-668-6

Prevention and Health: Directions for Policy and Practice

Prevention in Human Services
Volume 5, Number 1

CONTENTS

Introduction

This special issue is devoted to discussion of the prevention of health-related problems. Generally applied, prevention involves the use of all effective and practical means to reduce the incidence and prevalence of an illness or disease. There is much evidence that prevention works: many disorders can be avoided, their onset delayed, or their consequences mitigated.

Yet, health professionals and institutions are often justly criticized for devoting too much attention and money to curative programs, while downplaying or ignoring preventive activities. Government planners and policy-makers at all levels emphasize treatment intervention programs to the relative neglect of prevention efforts.

For all interested in health, including prevention specialists, this suggests that enhanced efforts must be made to ensure that the field of prevention takes its rightful place in the medical/psychiatric community. This requires that problem areas be more sharply defined, the incidence and prevalence of preventable disorders more clearly delineated, and more rigorous research conducted to test the impact of alternative prevention strategies and the cost-effectiveness of alternative approaches. Public relations/advocacy efforts must also be increased, since intelligent "marketing" strategies would heighten the visibility and acceptance of prevention activities. In line with such perspectives, this issue focuses on work being conducted in several important sectors of the health field.

In the Third World, high fertility levels are correlated with increased maternal and child morbidity/mortality patterns. In attempts to slow population growth, family planning programs aimed at birth prevention have been widely adopted. Ness and Landis explore the success of these national programs on a comparative basis, in terms of staffing, funding, political organization, and program inputs. The individual experiences of several countries are also examined.

The fourth leading cause of death in the United States is accidents. Of these, approximately 50% are attributed to motor vehicles. The Grant and McKinlay paper emphasizes the magnitude of the motor vehicle problem, discusses alternative solutions, and clarifies significant policy options. Seat belts, air bags, and trauma centers are among the modalities highlighted.

Among the chronic illnesses, asthma represents the leading cause of absenteeism in the schools. Asthma also involves high utilization of emergency medical care facilities, lowered self-esteem, and major life adjustments and restrictions. In the Weiss and Hermalin article, the first national study of a self-care pediatric asthma home-management program is discussed and evaluated. The program seeks to dispel myths about asthma, promote avoidance of asthma precipitants, clarify early warning signals, increase school attendance and self-esteem in young patients, and aid families and children in effectively managing the disorder. It is postulated that furthering this in-home, cost-effective program will reduce the need for emergency care and provide an important means of public education.

Development of effective strategies of immunization to ward off epidemic disease is, by its very nature, of concern not only to health planners and policy makers, but to the general community as well. Peterson compares the effects of diverse strategies in increasing immunization rates in the general population.

Infant nutrition by maternal breast-feeding as compared with the use of cow's milk formula products is a leading current concern in public health. The Jelliffes' paper reviews recent scientific findings that demonstrate the advantages of breast-feeding in nutrition, in the prevention of infant diseases and allergies, and as a natural factor in birth-spacing. These benefits are not limited to Third World societies, but apply also in the developed countries.

Richard Katz discusses the concept of the "synergistic community." He emphasizes the need to move away from a scarcity paradigm of goods and services to one based on constant community replenishment (synergism). While there are inequalities in the distribution of medical personnel, advanced technology, and treatment facilities, individuals can mobilize their talents and energies to provide ongoing support, assistance, and encouragement to one another. These opportunities have been neglected in the health field, and as with the "self-help" concept, warrant further exploration.

The ubiquitous concept of prevention has innumerable facets. It is the editors' hope that this special issue will be useful in illuminating some theoretical and practical aspects of health prevention.

Alfred H. Katz
Jared A. Hermalin
Robert E. Hess

Asian Family Planning: Observations in International Health and Birth Prevention Delivery Systems

Gayl D. Ness
Karl R. Landis
University of Michigan

SUMMARY. Rapid population growth in the Third World has been accompanied by the creation of national family planning programs, which attempt to slow growth rates through programs aimed at the prevention of births. These programs represent large scale, modern bureaucratic health delivery systems that are transplanted from the industrialized world. They raise the problem of whether such modern organizations can have an impact on reproductive behavior throughout the Third World. A large scale research program on Asian family planning programs provides some of the answers to these critical questions. First, pooled cross-national time series data indicate that as family planning programs grew and their inputs of staff and funds increased, both contraceptive and birth prevention increased. Further, multiple regression analyses indicate a positive impact of program inputs on both contraceptive use rates and birth prevention, even when levels of social and economic development are controlled. There is also, however, much variance among countries in their patterns of both program performance and birth prevention. Four country cases are examined—the Philippines, Malaysia, South Korea, and Indonesia—to show that the character of political organization has an impact on the performance of these modern bureaucratic birth prevention organizations.

The rapid growth of populations in the less developed countries constitutes a problem with wide implications. In addition to ecological pressures and economic costs, it is also a substantial health

The basic research reported here was supported by the US AID Office of Population, under contract number DPE-0632-C-00-1030-00. Requests for further information, data and reprints should be directed to the senior author, Gayl D. Ness, Department of Sociology, University of Michigan, Ann Arbor, MI 48109.

3

problem. Fertility is by no means pathological, but high fertility in a poor population can well be considered an epidemiological disease. High fertility typically implies that women bear children early, frequently and late in their reproductive lives. All three of these conditions are closely associated with high levels of maternal and child morbidity and mortality (Wray, 1972; Hobcraft, Mac-Donald & Rutstein, 1983; Population Reports, 1984).

The health problems associated with high fertility imply something almost counter-intuitive for the human community, namely that the promotion of family health is closely tied to the prevention of births. Of course, this notion does not apply to all births, but family health can be significantly improved by preventing (a) births among women under 20 and women over 35, (b) births at less than three year intervals, and (c) births of the third or higher order. Contemporary family planning programs among the less developed nations have focused their resources on the prevention of births that would fall into these three categories.

Throughout most of human history, governments have been pronatalist, so these highly focused birth prevention programs represent a major policy change for most governments. Never before have governments attempted to *prevent* births, especially within marriage, on such a wide scale. This policy change came about as government efforts to promote national economic development made decision-makers aware of the economic and family health costs of rapid population growth. The international community has joined in a large scale movement, currently mobilizing about half a billion dollars annually, to assist the governments of the less developed countries in their attempts to promote this specific type of birth prevention.

One of the most striking aspects of the new birth prevention efforts, however, is the enormous challenge they present to public health programming. This challenge raises many questions about the feasibility of such programming. Can large-scale, bureaucratic organizations effectively produce change in such a deeply ingrained aspect of human behavior? Also, can forms of organization and technology largely developed in the western world be used to promote the prevention of births in people of vastly different cultures, particularly among people afflicted with poverty, high levels of mortality, and low levels of literacy? It is clear that, especially among the less developed nations, birth prevention represents a major public health challenge.

This type of challenge has been faced before, of course. Smallpox, malaria, yaws, polio, and tetanus have all been effectively, if not completely, controlled through large-scale, bureaucratic disease prevention programs operating at both international and national levels. The birth prevention movement shows both differences and similarities to these other mass prevention programs. It differs in being far more controversial and tension ridden. Deep religious, ethnic, communal, or national sentiments that often supported disease prevention programs now stand as serious obstacles to the success of organized birth prevention programs. The birth prevention movement is similar to the disease prevention movements in organizational terms, since the determinants of effective service delivery in public health systems are of paramount concern to both.

Birth prevention, better known as family planning, programs are typically organized within a country's public health care delivery channels. The programs are usually controlled by health care professionals and are often located within national ministries of health. As a result, the organizational problems birth prevention programs face are similar to those of other public health or human service programs. However, the specific problems for the family planning programs center around the difficulty of creating a delivery system that can bring effective preventive services—education, information, and contraceptives—to a population that is burdened with a variety of poverty-related health problems and is often highly dispersed. Added problems stem from the international character of the movement, which involves the transfer of western medical technology across imposing cultural boundaries to environments where the patterns of kinship, the value of children, and the orientations to reproduction are quite different from those found in the industrialized countries. These cross-cultural transfers also entail organizational change as well. In the industrialized countries the technology of birth prevention flows largely through private market systems. In the less developed countries, this technology frequently moves through public health care systems, which are themselves bureaucratic transplants from a different culture.

These problems only raise more questions. Can these modern bureaucratic organizations move reproductive behavior in the direction of birth prevention? How can the effectiveness of these organizations be assessed? Do the programs vary in effectiveness, and if so, what determines the variance? Does the intrusion of the larger world community have an impact on this organized attempt to reduce fertility? More specifically, does foreign population assistance have any impact on the effectiveness of family planning programs?

We can examine some of these complex problems of national and international birth prevention by observing the general course of the Asian programs over the past two decades. For this examination we draw on the results of a research project of the University of Michigan's Center for Population Planning. This project collected most of the available data on 24 of the major countries in Asia, excluding Japan and China, for the period from 1950 to 1980. These data permit us to examine both the overall pattern of change in this large region, and the specific patterns of change within individual nations.

REGIONAL PATTERNS: ASIAN BIRTH PREVENTION, 1960-1980

The 24 major countries of Asia included in the study contained 1.5 billion people in 1980. Although some of the countries had no family planning program (Mongolia, North Korea, and Burma) and some of them had very little data (Kampuchea, Laos, and North Vietnam), 18 of the 24 countries did have programs, a portion of which had been in operation for almost two decades by 1980. By 1980, therefore, there was a total of 288 program years of experience from which statistical data could be obtained.

Figures 1 and 2 provide a rough approximation of the impact of this organized birth prevention activity, demonstrating that when births are being prevented in a high fertility society, the crude birth rate (births per thousand of the population) declines. Figure 1 shows a scattergram of the crude birth rates by the year of program duration. The negative slope of the regression line indicates that, as the Asian programs continued through time, the crude birth rate fell about half a point per year. In other words, as the programs continued through time, one birth was prevented each year for every two thousand people.

Figure 2 provides more direct evidence of the impact of the programs. It shows our estimate of the number of contraceptive users who receive their supplies from national family planning programs as a percent of all eligible couples by the year of program duration. In effect this shows the proportion of reproductive couples

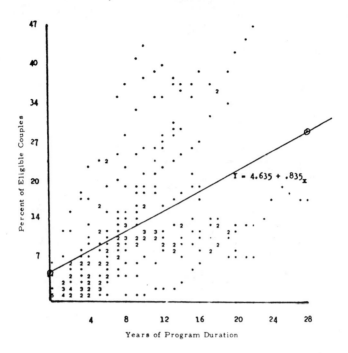

FIGURE 1. Crude Birth Rate by Family Planning Program
Duration for 19 Asian Countries (1952-1980).

who are using program-supplied contraceptives in deliberate attempts to prevent births. This scatterplot also shows that as the
Asian programs progressed through time, there was an increase of
almost 0.9 percentage points per year in deliberate birth preventors.

These scattergrams provide only a rough approximation of
program performance, of course, in part because there is spread
around the regression lines. Later we shall deal with this spread by
examining variance in individual country program performance.
Further, they suggest only an *association,* not causation, between
program operation and deliberate birth prevention. Determining
causation requires more specific observations.

One of the ways to address the issue of causation is to enter the
debate that has gone on in social demography over the relative
impact of socio-economic (SE) changes and family planning program efforts in producing fertility limitation through individual
prevention of births. Compelling evidence suggests that people

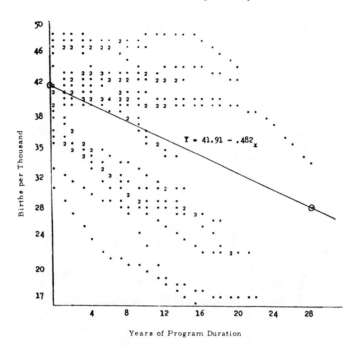

FIGURE 2. Program-Supplied Contraceptive Users by Years of
Program Duration for 19 Asian Countries (1952 - 1980).

generally begin to limit their fertility when social and economic
conditions improve substantially and consistently (Mauldin &
Berelson, 1978; Hernandez, 1981; Cutwright, 1984). We have
already seen in Figures 1 and 2 that the operation of family planning
programs is also associated with birth prevention. The important
question, whether this association is independent of changes in
fertility caused by the socio-economic conditions, remains, but can
be addressed through the construction of a series of multiple
regression equations.

First, Table 1 shows the simple correlation coefficients between
the Crude Birth Rate (CBR), a measure of birth prevention, and a
variety of measures of socio-economic development and family
planning program operations. We have used a standard set of
indicators, with gross domestic product (GDP) per capita as a
measure of the wealth or productivity of a country, life expectancy
at birth (E_0) and infant mortality rate (IMR) as measures of health,
and literacy as a measure of social development. We have used one

Table 1.
Correlation Coefficients Between Measures
of Socioeconomic Change, Family Planning
Programs Inputs and Outputs, and Crude Birth Rate
for Asia 1960-1980.†

Variable	Correlation Coefficients for: (Ns for each coefficient are shown in parentheses)						
	CBR	GDP/cap	E_o	IMR	Literacy	Contraceptive Users	FP Staff
GDP/cap	-.682 (426)						
E_o	-.863 (494)	.691 (435)					
IMR	.835 (486)	-.622 (426)	-.956 (498)				
Literacy	-.673 (466)	.440 (439)	.810 (462)	-.825 (460)			
Contraceptive Users	-.591 (274)	.541 (270)	.548 (281)	-.561 (271)	.526 (275)		
F.P.Staff	.083 (162)	-.151 (161)	-.015 (162)	-.004 (162)	.085 (162)	.267 (160)	
Gov't FP Expenditures	-.308 (218)	.618 (215)	.360 (221)	-.376 (217)	.358 (221)	.475 (208)	.046 (153)

NB. Prevalence (users) data are in percent of eligible couples; staff, and expenditure data are per 1,000 eligible couples.

†These correlations represent the relationships for 24 Asian countries between 1960 and 1980 with each year acting as a point of observation.

9

output measure for the birth prevention programs, contraceptive users as a percentage of eligible couples, and two input measures, family planning staff and government expenditures—both per thousand eligible couples. Note first that all of the relationships are in the predicted direction: as wealth, life expectancy, and literacy rise, more births are prevented; as infant mortality declines, more births are prevented; as family planning inputs increase, outputs increase; and as outputs increase, more births are prevented.

We have also tested a series of models with multiple regression equations for these data. The models reflect our notions about causation and are stated with sufficient specificity to permit their test with statistical manipulations. We present two significant equations here as summaries of our tests. The first equation indicates that, in Asia, increases in *both* life expectancy (a surrogate measure of all socio-economic development), and contraceptive use lead to a decline in fertility, i.e., an increase in birth prevention. Regression analysis allows us to conclude that each factor has an independent impact on birth prevention. These findings support the argument that organized, bureaucratic prevention programs can have the same type of preventive impact on reproductive behavior as they have had on major infectious diseases.

$$
\begin{aligned}
Y(\text{CBR}) &= -.832(\text{E}_\text{o}) - .139(\% \text{ users}) \\
(\text{SE}) &= (.029) \qquad\quad (.029) \\
R^2 &= .84,\ p < .001
\end{aligned}
$$

The second equation addresses the question of the sources of programs effectiveness, i.e., what permits the programs to produce the desired outputs. This equation uses program outputs, contraceptive users, as the dependent variable. It indicates that three things each have a significant, independent impact on this output. The first factor is literacy, which is a surrogate measure for a more general condition of social development, but the other two are simple program inputs: money and staff. Therefore, even when we controlled for literacy, the more staff and money Asian governments expend on their family planning programs, the higher the number of people recruited for deliberate birth preventive behavior.

$$
\begin{aligned}
Y(\% \text{ users}) &= .334(\text{lit}) + .235(\text{staff}) + .338(\text{exp}) \\
(\text{SE}) &= (.070) \qquad\quad (.067) \qquad\quad (.070) \\
R^2 &= .36,\ p < .001
\end{aligned}
$$

The Asian experience is thus somewhat reassuring to those who construct large-scale, preventive, public health programs, even in such sensitive areas as reproduction. It indicates that, independently of the substantial socio-economic changes Asian countries have experienced over the past two decades, investing money and staff in family planning programs did produce a substantial increase in the deliberate use of birth preventive actions.

If all of Asia in summary showed this positive experience, it is also clear that some birth prevention programs were much more effective than others in achieving their ends. For instance, programs in South Korea, Taiwan, Thailand, and Indonesia have been very successful in promoting birth prevention, while Pakistan and Bangladesh have had many years of program experience with virtually no success. These country-specific histories of program efficiency can be expressed in terms of output-input ratios. In other words, in South Korea, Taiwan, Thailand, and Indonesia, staff and money inputs into birth prevention programs have led to substantial outputs both in terms of the number of people recruited as new acceptors of contraception per staff member per year, and in terms of the percentage of people who are actively trying to prevent births (contraceptive users). In Pakistan and Bangladesh, however, continuing large inputs have not led to these program outputs. These ratios prove to be useful mechanisms for examining program performance with greater precision, since we can use them to capture varying levels of program performance.

Before proceeding, let us describe the two output-input ratios in more detail. The first is the number of contraceptive *acceptors* recruited per program staff member each year. The second is the number of continuing contraceptive *users* in the population per staff member in any year.[1] Often prevention programs that rely on individual action must recruit people to the desired behavior, and then assure that those initially recruited continue to act in support of that prevention. For example, to prevent the gastro-intestinal diseases that are widespread killers of children in poor countries, there must be an initial recruitment of mothers to teach them such things as oral rehydration therapy. Then there must be continuing care in feeding to achieve success. For mass prevention programs then, it is possible to assess program effectiveness by assessing both the *new recruitment*, and the *continued use* achieved per unit of program inputs.

The first question to ask of these output-input ratios is how they change over the duration of a program. Our reasoning about family planning programs would predict that a new program should have relatively high levels of acceptors and users per input, since it taps a demand for assistance that remained relatively unmet prior to the program's inception. Then, as the program progresses through time, it will meet greater resistance once it exhausts the initial demand and begins to meet what many have called the hard core of high fertility people. This hypothesis anticipates a negative slope of efficiency, or output-to-input ratio, over the life of the program.

The following equations show that this picture is only partly accurate. The first equation shows that for Asian programs overall, recruitment efficiency (r.eff) has indeed declined over the lives of the programs. On the average, in each year of program life, 4.3 fewer acceptors are recruited per staff member than the year before. On the other hand, the second equation shows that user efficiency (u.eff) increased over the lives of the programs, although this increase is not statistically significant. In regression analysis with one predictor variable, a nonsignificant equation means the increase or decrease is within the bounds of sampling fluctuation, and is therefore not statistically distinguishable from a horizontal line with no slope. Thus, while it appears that staff effectiveness in recruiting acceptors declines slightly over time, staff effectiveness in gaining and maintaining contraceptive users does not decline and may even rise over time. Although we do not show the equations, we have found the same relationships when we consider the cost of recruiting new acceptors and the cost of maintaining contraceptive users. The overall cost per new acceptor rises about $.85 (U.S.) per year, but the cost per user remains stable. These data are recorded in current prices, not adjusted for inflation; therefore, since all countries experienced substantial inflation during this period, the *real* costs for both recruiting new acceptors and maintaining users must actually have declined over time.

$$Y(\text{r.eff}) = 179 - 4.3(\text{program duration}) \ R^2 = .05, p < .003$$
$$Y(\text{u.eff}) = 188 + 2.6(\text{program duration}) \ R^2 = .00, p < .26$$

These findings provide a picture of birth prevention programs that has not yet been considered in the literature on program performance. While most of that literature has considered costs in terms of annual operations, our findings demonstrate that the time dimension adds an important insight. Each year program inputs generate immediate outputs in the form of new acceptors, but those inputs also generate contraceptive users for subsequent years. In other words, a full consideration of birth prevention program costs should discount annual costs to reflect the returns a program generates for future years. No attempt has yet been made to estimate either what that discount rate should be, or to what extent it should reduce the projected costs of a program in its inception.

We can now investigate other conditions which may affect program efficiency. Our study considered a wide range of conditions, but we will merely summarize the most salient findings here, focusing on the socio-economic environment, the political environment, and foreign assistance. In all cases we have used the multiple regression techniques shown above, but we present the findings in a simpler narrative form.

The first condition to be considered is the socio-economic environment. Clearly, if rising socioeconomic conditions lead individuals to prevent births on their own, this condition will also be associated with higher levels of program efficiency. For example, it will be easier to explain the health benefits of birth prevention to educated women than to illiterate women. This explanation will also be easier when women believe that their children will live than it will when women experience frequent infant and child deaths. As expected, we found that the socioeconomic environment is highly related to both measures of program efficiency; therefore, in subsequent analyses we controlled for the socioeconomic environment when examining other determinants of efficiency.

What conditions beyond general socioeconomic development affect program performance? The literature on the politics of development can be useful here, since these birth prevention programs are like many other human-service development programs. From Edward Shills's (1960) early treatment of development in general to Pai Panandiker's (1978) more recent treatment of India, the development literature has argued that political and administrative conditions have a great impact on the performance of all types of development programs. A strong political center is needed to make difficult decisions on the priorities of resource allocation and to drive the administration to high levels of goal achievement. There has also been a great deal of discussion of the importance of the "political will" or "political commitment" of the top leadership for the success of birth prevention programs. Inaddition, the general literature suggests that higher levels of administrative decentralization and local participation facilitate program performance, because this permits general aims and techniques to be adapted to the unique conditions of any local situation. Further, decentralization tends to increase local initiative, thus giving programs active leadership at all levels.

We have measured both central political strength[2] and administrative decentralization for all countries through the entire three decades, and our data generally support the arguments found in the development literature. We found that recruitment efficiency is positively associated both with the degree of central political strength and with the degree of political and administrative decentralization. User efficiency, or continuation, on the other hand, is not affected by the degree of political centralization, although it is positively affected by the degree of administrative decentralization and local participation. This suggests that in the initiation of a birth prevention program, and in the organization of an efficient program, a strong central government is important. On the other hand, increasing the program's effectiveness in maintaining contraceptive users requires more initiative and participation at local levels.

Another condition that may affect program efficiency is international assistance. About a dozen major donor nations in the industrialized world now provide more than half a billion dollars yearly for this type of technical assistance, but we find that the volume of this assistance has no impact on program efficiency. Adding donor assistance, either in total or from any of the individual donors, to our multiple regression equations does not add to the explanatory power of socio-economic and political conditions. As with the political conditions, this finding is consistent with our knowledge of individual country program histories. Pakistan, Bangladesh, and the Philippines have all received large amounts of foreign assistance, yet all of these programs show little success. Taiwan has received very little assistance, yet it shows considerable success. Thailand and Indonesia show both large amounts of assistance and high levels of program success. The simple volume of aid does not appear to affect program efficiency. We shall see below, however, that some of the less quantifiable characteristics of foreign assistance can be quite effective in helping programs to become more efficient.

INDIVIDUAL COUNTRY EXPERIENCES

As we saw in Figures 1 and 2, the summary statements of all Asian programs taken together hide much individual country variance in the public promotion of birth prevention. We can only illustrate this variance here by discussing several cases that will outline its range. We will use the histories of programs in the Philippines, Malaysia, South Korea, and Indonesia for this illustration. In each case, we examine the role of political conditions and the role of foreign assistance in the national birth prevention program. This follows our earlier statistical analyses of the pan-Asian experience. While we used simple quantitative indicators of political and foreign aid conditions in the multiple regression analyses, the case studies permit us to deal with the richer, more qualitative conditions that affect this type of public prevention programming. To provide some statistical base for the illustrations, for each country we show the movement of both newly recruited acceptors per staff (recruiting efficiency) and the current contraceptive users (total output of continuing prevention) for each year of the program.

The Philippines

The Philippines (Figures 3 and 4) shows the most erratic behavior over time. The number of contraceptive users (Figure 3) grew rapidly during the first few years of the program then declined for roughly the last half of its life. Recruitment efficiency (Figure 4) maintained a roughly steady level, it first rose rapidly about 1976, then dropped equally rapidly and rose again.

The most pervasive condition that might affect program performance in the Philippines is, of course, religion. As the only Roman Catholic country in the region, Philippine birth prevention is restrained by ambivalence on the part of the ruling elite, i.e., political resistance, to a national family planning program. Although the Church has been something of a silent partner in Philippines population planning (Ness, 1982), it has also provided important points of resistance to the program. The Council of Bishops was persuaded to accept, or to refrain from public opposition to, family planning by the creation of a ''Responsible Parenthood Program'' which promoted the use of the rhythm method. Nevertheless, there has been considerable conflict within the church

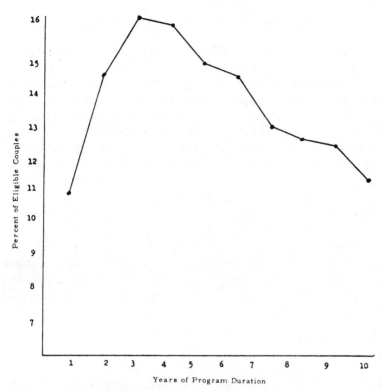

FIGURE 3. Phillippines: Program-Supplied Contraceptive
Users by Years of Program Duration.

over family planning (Gorospe, 1970), and the opposition of
specific top bureaucrats and political leaders also reflects an
ambivalent stance toward these programs.

Less visible, but perhaps more important in the Philippines, is a
weak and over-centralized political-administrative system, which
appears far more effective in directing resources to national leaders
than in achieving the stated goals of any public program (Ness,
1982). The national family planning program began in 1970 with a
top level coordinating board, the Population Commission. It was
first committed to the development of a careful and fully professional clinical medical program, which necessarily restricted services to the more urbanized population. Only after considerable
pressure did the government move services beyond the clinics to the
more dispersed and inaccessible rural population. The overall

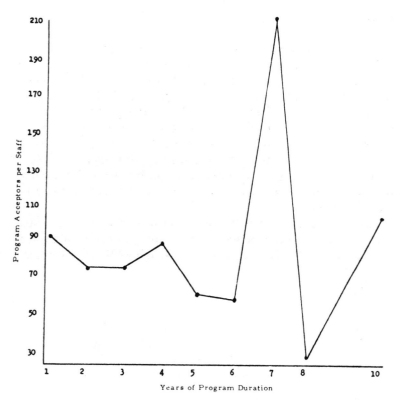

FIGURE 4. Philippines: Family Planning Program Acceptors
per Staff by Years of Program Duration.

administrative condition of the program has been judged weak by a
number of external observers (Health Services Report, 1977), and
this weakness is perhaps best illustrated by the program's internal
accounting procedures. Although the program has centralized computer capacities, it is exceptionally weak in field controls for data
collection. For many years this led program managers to simply
reduce the reported output of all units of the program by 20 percent.

The weakness of the Philippines program is not related to foreign
assistance, since it has received the highest per capita levels of
foreign assistance of any country in Asia.[3] However, the millions of
dollars of foreign aid received by the Philippines have not had any
appreciable impact on the effectiveness of the birth prevention
programs.

Malaysia

Figures 5 and 6 show continuing users and recruitment efficiency ratios for Malaysia over the life of its national family planning program. Use has risen, although with some erratic drops (Figure 5). More dramatic, however, is the consistent decline in program efficiency over time (Figure 6). Unlike the Philippines, Malaysia is judged to have a strong and generally efficient political-administrative system (Ness, 1967; Ness & Ando, 1971). Its birth prevention program resulted from its own very successful internal quest for national social and economic development, but the birth prevention program has never been as successful nor as efficient as Malaysia's other ventures.

Observers familiar with Malaysian history recognize the importance of the delicate ethnic balance for explaining almost all program and political dynamics. With roughly 50 percent Malayʳ

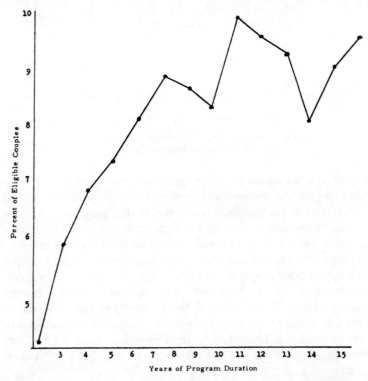

FIGURE 5. Malaysia: Program-Supplied Contraceptive Users by Years of Program Duration.

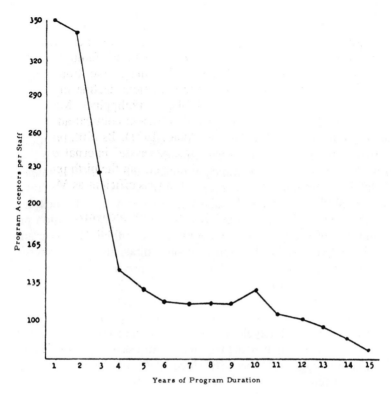

FIGURE 6. Malaysia: Family Planning Program Acceptors
per Staff by Years of Program Duration.

40 percent Chinese, and 10 percent Indians, Malaysia's ethnic
balance is unstable and requires extremely sensitive leadership. The
series of bloody racial clashes in the post-war period attest to the
volatility of the underlying conflicts. If population policies often
give rise to deep-seated conflicts, they do so almost inevitably when
the country is ethnically divided.

It is instructive to note that Malaysia made its initial birth prevention policy decision in 1964-6, just after the government won
overwhelming victories in the polls, producing a degree of popular
support and confidence that the national leadership has not known
since. The program went into the field in 1966/67 and grew rapidly
for two years. Then the country was rocked, in 1969, by some of the
most violent racial strife it has known since the end of World War
II. The conflict erupted when the ruling party lost its majority in two

critical states: Selangor and Perak. An emergency was declared, parliament was closed, and the country was ruled by a national emergency council under martial law for almost two years. One result of this violence was a policy to reduce the visibility and vigor of the national family planning program and to reinforce the ethnic-based ambivalence about population planning that had lain dormant when the government felt strong and confident. More recently Malaysia has taken an even more dramatic turn, as the Prime Minister announced in the summer of 1982 that the country should aim to increase its population from the current 13 million to 70 million! There is little doubt in the minds of most observers that the intent is to increase the number and proportion of Malays, i.e., to further outnumber the Chinese and Indians. These events clearly show how government strength, or popularity, supports birth prevention programming, while government weakness undermines the program.

The external world has intruded only modestly into Malaysian population or development affairs. The country is wealthy and well organized, and has been able to mobilize with ease the capital it needs for development. It has, to be sure, received large World Bank loans, with substantial monies for population planning included in the overall development packages the bank provides. Still, it is difficult to argue that these loans are essential to Malaysia's population program, especially since many of the allotted funds have not been used.

South Korea

South Korea has one of the older programs in the region, set in a country that claims distinction for its miracle of development. The progression of users and the recruitment efficiency ratio for South Korea are seen in Figures 7 and 8. Use has risen steadily (Figure 7). Program efficiency has also risen, but less steadily, and has shown a slight downturn at the end of the 1970s (Figure 8). Like Malaysia, Korea's policy decision came out of its own internal social and economic planning, and out of the health care delivery problems that resulted from rapid population growth by the early 1960s. Korea's program is especially interesting because of its early use of the IUD, which demands good clinical and outreach services, but also provides high levels of protection for the recruitment of acceptors. Even today, when most programs make heavy, if not exclusive, use of the contraceptive pill, South Korea continues to show substantial propor-

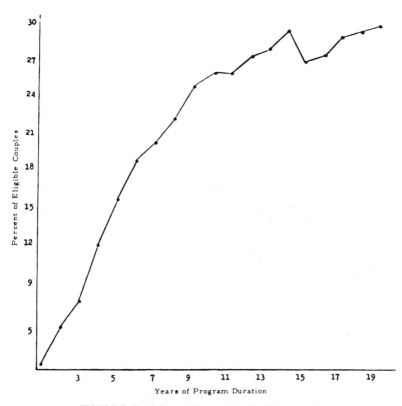

FIGURE 7. South Korea: Program-Supplied Contraceptive
Users by Years of Program Duration.

tions of acceptors using the IUD, and increasing proportions using
sterilization.

Korea's alleged economic miracle has involved a broad-based
development program in which rapid growth has been accompanied
by equality in the distribution of wealth. It has also included a heavy
emphasis on education and health as part of the human services
offered extensively to both rural and urban populations. In effect, the
family planning program is merely one of a number of effectively
managed human service programs that raise the level of welfare along
with human productivity. The downturns in efficiency at the end of
the 1970s may simply reflect the successes of development programming. This implies that the population will be increasingly well
served by a private market, and that the family planning program will
be less and less an exclusive mechanism for providing contraceptive

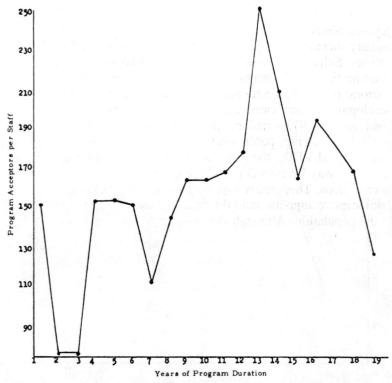

FIGURE 8. South Korea: Family Planning Acceptors per Staff by Years of Program Duration.

services. This may also raise program costs, since those well served by the private market will tend to be the more urban population, leaving the national family planning program with the costly task of serving the more dispersed rural population.

Indonesia

Our final example is Indonesia. It is both the largest and the poorest of the four countries considered here. Its poverty, size, and great population dispersion would not normally lead to the prediction of a successful family planning program, yet it has become well known for its striking successes (Hull, Hull & Singarimbun, 1977). Figures 9 and 10 show the strong rise in both continuing use and recruitment efficiency ratios over the lifetime of the program.

Indonesia's political history is remarkable for its total reversal from the anti-development and pronatalist policy stance under

President Sukarno. The coup, with its bloody aftermath in 1965-6, deposed Sukarno and brought General Suharto to rule as a virtual military dictator. The change of leaders also brought a change of policies. Suharto reinstated the technocrats who had gone into exile or domestic oblivion under Sukarno, and he started the country on a strong program of national economic development. Out of this development effort came a strong antinatalist policy decision in 1968, and by 1972 a national program was in the field through the small, but growing, public health system.

In the mid-1970s, the program underwent an important change, breaking away from its clinical base of operations to a village base of operations. This greatly expanded the service outlets and brought contraceptive supplies and information to a much larger proportion of the population. Although this program change was initiated and

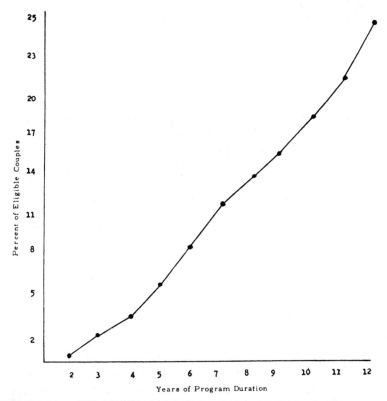

FIGURE 9. Indonesia: Program-Supplied Contraceptive Users by Years of Program Duration.

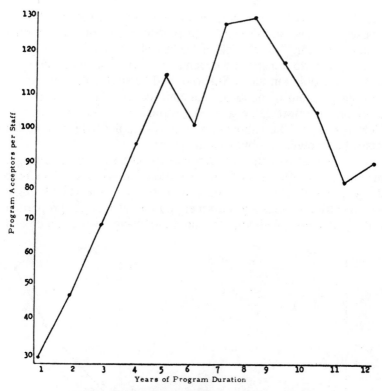

FIGURE 10. Indonesia: Family Planning Program Acceptors
per Staff by Years of Program Duration.

directed by Indonesians, it was greatly expedited by the US AID
Population Office, which provided some of the most effective foreign
assistance to be found in the history of international population
assistance (Heiby, Ness & Pillsbury 1979). US AID provided substantial grants to the Indonesian program, but it was probably more
important for the process of service delivery than for the amount of
funds it granted. AID officers, together with their Indonesian counterparts developed a mechanism for moving funds rapidly from the
capital to provincial and district offices. This helped to stimulate a
high level of local initiative which, in turn, helped to adapt the
general program organization to specific local conditions.

One other general set of environmental conditions has undoubtedly helped Indonesia to maintain steady growth in its program.
Since 1950, the country has made sustained progress in the spread

of education, especially to the rural areas and the outer provinces. Rates of literacy and school attendance have risen rapidly and have become nearly equal for males and females. In addition, Indonesia has built a series of provincial medical schools which produce a large cadre of medical professionals appropriately trained for rural health services. The country has been able to extract a compulsory two to three years of service in rural clinics from these medical graduates. Both developments are symptomatic of an administrative decentralization that has stressed the development of rural and provincial initiative. In addition, the high degree of political centralization under the military rule, and the relatively high administrative decentralization that characterize the country provide conditions that support rather than suppress program development.

CONCLUSIONS

The population problem in Asia has attracted world attention for the better part of this century. It has also attracted the attention of Asian planners who have provided important leadership in moving toward national policies of birth prevention through the distribution of modern contraceptives. Even before the United Nations was willing to discuss problems of rapid population growth, India, Sri Lanka, and Pakistan made their own policy decisions to work toward birth prevention. Today, therefore, Asia presents the world with the longest, richest, and most fully documented set of national programs deliberately designed to prevent births.

Although the motivations for these programs have been mixed, two aims in particular have remained dominant. One is the aim of national economic development, the achievement of which was seen to be obstructed by rapid population growth. The second is individual health and welfare. It has long been recognized that bearing children either early, frequently, or late in the reproductive life cycle is detrimental to maternal and child health. Thus one of the aims of the national family planning programs has been preventive in character. These programs have aimed to prevent death and sickness by changing the patterns of childbearing that are important causes of death and sickness.

This long history of family planning programs also provides us with the opportunity to assess the effectiveness of modern preventive health programs. Family planning in Asia is essentially a modern bureaucratic activity in which large-scale organizations attempt to prevent births by distributing modern contraceptive information and supplies. The Asian experience has permitted us to ask whether these bureaucratically organized national programs can be effective in changing something as profound as human reproductive behavior. Although our data do not provide conclusive answers to all these questions, they can be used to make some important observations.

First, deliberate birth prevention has produced fertility decline in Asia, although with varying success. Taiwan, South Korea, Hong Kong, Singapore, Fiji, Thailand, Indonesia, and Sri Lanka have all experienced substantial fertility decline. The declines have been more moderate in India, Pakistan, and Malaysia. Iran does not appear to have experienced any real fertility decline, nor have Afghanistan or Bangladesh.

Second, the effectiveness of these birth prevention programs is clearly associated with the type of social and economic changes that occur in each country. In the multiple regression equations our data permit, both the socioeconomic conditions and the program outputs contribute significantly to birth prevention. Equally important are the observations that the inputs into family planning programs, both staff and funds, contribute significantly to the program outputs. Although these data cannot be said to prove the point, they do support the proposition that modern family planning programs can be rationally constructed to have a preventive impact on reproductive behavior. Although bureaucratic instruments are being transplanted from one set of cultures to another, and although these instruments are being used to distribute an equally foreign technology to populations with vastly different and deeply rooted value systems, it does appear that this type of rational organization can be effective.

Our data suggest that this particular rational bureaucratic action will be more effective where the social and economic environment is more developed. This makes intuitive sense, because more advanced social and economic conditions imply that a government has access to more human and financial resources, more funds for the budget, and more literate people to choose from for whatever public program it adopts. However, it is not only the diffuse social and economic resource level that appears to affect the performance of public birth preventive programs. A strong political center and a high degree of political and administrative centralization appear to facilitate program performance as well. We suggest that the strong center is needed to mobilize resources for the program, both to establish goals for and demand high performance from the programs for which it mobilizes resources. Decentralization is thought to facilitate program performance by permitting a more sensitive adaptation of a technology to varying local conditions.

Finally, our data suggest that, for the region as a whole, neither the absolute level of foreign assistance funds, nor the pattern of sources, has a direct and consistent impact on either program outputs or program performance, as measured by output-input ratios. The histories of the individual countries suggest, however, that while foreign aid may be important, it is never decisive. It cannot create or sustain an effective program where local political-administrative commitments and capacities are lacking. If, however, a national leadership is strongly committed to effective public programming, sensitively directed foreign aid can provide substantial assistance, especially where the level of economic development is low and domestic financial resources tend to be strained. Our own field experience suggests that foreign assistance channelled through a technically and culturally competent field operation can be especially helpful in providing effective foreign aid for birth prevention. We have seen programs like this in Indonesia, Thailand, South Korea, and especially in Taiwan.

Thus the long and rich history of national family planning or birth prevention programs in Asia provides evidence that programs *can* be effective in changing even deeply embedded behaviors such as those that govern reproduction. In being effective in this area, these human service programs can also have a substantial impact on both individual and societal health.

NOTES

1. The user output-input ratio is unique from that for the acceptors recruited because the different contraceptive technologies vary in the duration of effect. For example, sterilization yields a contraceptive user for life, whereas birth control pills yield a user only for the duration of the supply of pills dispensed.

2. Central political strength is assessed through a narrative scale indicating the strength of a ruling party or group and its control over the territory of the state. Political and administrative decentralization is assessed through a narrative scale that gives higher points for systems that permit and experience organized political opposition and that show substantial decentralization of authority and responsibility in the administrative system. In all cases, these political conditions are assessed by a coding system that used multiple coders so intercoder reliability could be assessed.

3. Total foreign assistance in U.S. dollars rose from $38,000 in 1960 to $15.6 million in 1980, for a per 100 population increase of $0.14 to $32.

REFERENCES

Berelson, B. & Ronald, F. (1976). Family planning programs: Where we stand. *Studies in Family Planning, 7,* 1-40.

Blake, J. (1982). Sociological perspectives on population studies. *Population Theory and Policy.* Urbana-Champaign & Chicago: University of Chicago Press.

Cutwright, P. (1983). The ingredients of recent fertility decline in developing countries. *International Family Planning Perspectives, 9,* 101-109.

Family Health Services, Inc. (1977). *A review of the Philippines population program.* Washington, DC: Family Health Services, Inc.

Gorospe, V. R. (ed.) (1970). *Responsible parenthood in the Philippines.* Manila: Ateneo University.

Heiby, J., Ness, G. D. & Pillsbury, B. (1979). *AID's role in Indonesian family planning.* Washington, DC: USAID, Bureau of Policy Planning and Coordination.

Hernandez, D. J. (1981). The impact of family planning programs on fertility: A critical evaluation. *Social Science Research, 10,* 32-66.

Hobcraft, J., MacDonald, J. W. & Rutstein, R. (1983). Child spacing effects on early child mortality. *Population Index, 49,* 585-618.

Hull, T., Hull, V. & Singarimbun, M. (1977). Indonesia's family planning story: Success and challenge. *Population Bulletin.*

Lynch, F. (1978). *The church: Silent partner in Philippines population planning.* Unpublished manuscript.

Mauldin, W. P. & Berelson, B. (1978). The conditions of fertility decline in developing countries. *Studies in Family Planning, 9,* 90-148.

Morris, M. D. (1979). *Measuring the condition of the world's poor: The physical quality of life index.* Washington, DC: Overseas Development Council.

Ness, G. D. (1967). *Bureaucracy and rural development in Malaysia.* Berkeley: University of California Press.

Ness, G. D. & Ando, H. (1971). The politics of population planning in Malaysia and the Philippines. *Journal of Comparative Administration, 3,* 296-329.

Ness, G. D. (1982). Philippines population planning: Some provocative observations. In George Foriol (ed.), *Population and security in the Philippines.* Washington, DC: Georgetown University Center for Strategic and International Studies.

Ness, G. D., Johnson, T. J. & Bernstein, S. (1983). *Asian family planning program performance.* Ann Arbor: University of Michigan Center for Population Planning.

Ness, G. D. & Ando, H. (1984). *The land is shrinking: Population planning in Asia.* Baltimore: Johns Hopkins University Press.

Pai Panandiker, V. A. (1978). *Bureaucracy and development administration.* New Delhi: Center for Policy Research.

Shils, E. (1960). Political development in the new states. *Comparative Studies in Society and History, 2,* 265-92 & 379-411.

Wray, J. W. (1972). *Population pressure on families: Family size and child spacing.* Baltimore: Johns Hopkins University Press.

Appropriate Technology
Applied to a Western Epidemic:
The Case of Motor Vehicle Accidents

Karen R. Grant
Boston University

John B. McKinlay
Boston University
Cambridge Research Center/
American Institutes for Research

SUMMARY. The fourth leading cause of death in the United States is accidents. Of these, about one-half are attributed to motor vehicle accidents. This paper emphasizes the magnitude of the problem, discusses possible solutions, and clarifies significant policy options. Seat belts, air bags, and trauma units are among the options highlighted.

In America today, accidents remain the fourth leading cause of death, with this country's youth being especially vulnerable. Nearly half of such accidents are the result of motor vehicle crashes, with results seen by some analysts as a national tragedy. No clear or rational public health policy has emerged to deal with the problem of motor vehicle accidents (MVAs) despite the fact that the mortality and morbidity associated with MVAs are largely preventable. Other countries, such as Canada, Great Britain and Australia, have successfully brought injuries and deaths from MVAs under control through legislation mandating seat belt usage. In America, however, there has been adamant resistance to such legislation. Instead, there has been a burgeoning of medical facilities to provide emergency medical care (trauma centers) to respond to the problem of MVAs.

This research was supported in part by the National Health Research and Development Program (Health and Welfare, Canada) through a National Health Fellowship (# 6607-1374-47) and by a Social Science and Humanities Research Council of Canada Doctoral Fellowship (# 453-83-0366) to the first author. Reprints may be obtained from Karen R. Grant, Department of Sociology, University of Manitoba, Winnipeg, Manitoba, Canada R3T 2N2.

While these centers have substantially improved accident victims' chances of survival, the efficacy and appropriateness of this intervention remains open to question. Rather than promoting a preventive health policy, our infatuation with and belief in medical technology has led to this post-hoc palliative intervention (a logical extension of the allopathic model of medicine), which provides a superficial, short-term response to the problem, without actually reducing it.

Researchers looking at the problems of the developing world often claim that as the challenges faced by these countries are largely environmental and preventable, they can best be resolved through a health policy premised on the notion of primary care which includes, but is not restricted to, the deployment of "appropriate technology" (International Conference on Primary Care, 1978). It is now apparent that this type of health policy has considerable relevance in the developed world, whose health problems are also primarily environmental and preventable.

This paper examines the alarming problem of MVAs in America today, with particular attention to policies designed to ameliorate this problem. The discussion is divided into three parts. *First*, we identify the magnitude of the problem, noting the nature and distribution of traffic injuries and fatalities. *Second*, we employ concepts from the political economy of health and illness and the sociology of development to describe viable ways of dealing with the epidemic of MVA injury and death. And *finally*, the paper closes with a discussion of major policy options.

THE EPIDEMIC OF MOTOR VEHICLE ACCIDENTS

In *The Politics of Cancer*, Samuel Epstein made the following observation:

> If one thousand people died every day of cholera, swine flu, or food poisoning, an epidemic of major proportions would be at hand and the entire community would mobilize against it. Yet cancer claims that many lives daily, often in prolonged and agonizing pain, and most people believe they can do nothing about it. Cancer, they think, strikes where it will, with no apparent cause. . . . But cancer has distinct, identifiable causes. It is not just another degenerative disease associated

with aging. It can be largely prevented. . . . The control and prevention of cancer will require a concerted national effort. (1978, p. 1).

Although some (Douglas & Wildavsky, 1982) question Epstein's claims, the environmental component in cancer etiology is beyond dispute, as is the fact that the probability of developing cancer in the modern era seems ominously high.

A somewhat analogous situation is presented by motor vehicle-related fatalities and injuries in the United States. Evidence from many different sources reveals the epidemic proportions of death and injury due to MVAs (e.g., the U.S. National Center for Health Statistics, the U.S. National Highway Traffic Safety Administration [NHTSA], and the National Safety Council) (Haddon, 1980). Accidental death (motor vehicle and other) is the fourth major cause of death, preceded only by coronary heart disease, cancer, and cerebrovascular incidents; it has retained that position since the 1950s (Fingerhut, Wilson & Feldman, 1980). MVA-related fatalities fall disproportionately on young people.

Although customarily used to describe an acute outbreak of *infectious* disease (e.g., the plague, cholera, etc.), the modern usage of "epidemics" applies equally well to noninfectious problems characterized by excessive prevalence (MacMahon & Pugh, 1970). Put another way, "an epidemic, or outbreak, is the occurrence of a disease in members of a defined population clearly in excess of the number of cases usually or normally found in that population" (Friedman, 1980, p. 73; cf. Last, 1983).

Table 1 presents the leading causes of death in the United States since 1960. There has been a decline in mortality from all causes, and among the leading causes of death, the most dramatic reductions are from the cardiovascular diseases, for reasons which are not yet clear. While malignant neo-plasms continue taking more lives, deaths from all accidents evidence some decline. A disturbing pattern is evident with respect to MVA mortality, however. In 1960, there were 11.4 million MVAs in America which resulted in 38,100 deaths (within one year of the accidents). By 1972, there was a peak in the total number of deaths from MVAs, resulting in some 56,528 fatalities (Tables 2 and 3). A reduction in deaths from MVAs was observed from 1973 through 1977, after which there was a sustained increase. In 1980, close to 52,000 people died in MVAs, represent-

TABLE 1

Death Rates, 1960 to 1979, and Deaths, 1970 to 1979,

From Selected Causes

	All Causes	Major Cardio-vascular Diseases*	Malig-nancies	Accidents & Adverse Effects	Motor Vehicle Accidents**
CRUDE DEATH RATES PER 100,000 POP.					
1960	954.7	515.1	149.2	52.3	21.3
1970	945.3	496.0	162.8	56.4	26.9
1975	888.5	455.8	171.7	48.4	21.5
1978	883.4	442.7	181.9	48.4	24.0
1979	869.5	435.4	183.9	47.8	24.3
AGE ADJUSTED DEATH RATES PER 100,000 POP.***					
1970	714.3	340.1	129.9	53.7	27.4
1975	638.3	291.4	130.9	44.8	21.3
1979	588.8	259.3	133.2	43.7	23.7
DEATHS (1,000)					
1970	1921.0	1008.0	330.7	114.6	54.6
1975	1892.9	971.0	365.7	103.0	45.9
1979	1913.8	958.3	403.4	105.3	53.5

*Includes deaths from cerebrovascular diseases.

**"Motor Vehicle Accidents" is a sub-category of "Accidents and Adverse Effects".

***Based on resident population enumerated as of April 1 for 1960 and 1970, and estimated as of July 1 for other years.

Source: Statistical Abstract of the United States, 1982-83, 1982, p. 76 (based on U.S. National Center for Health Statistics, Vital Statistics of the United States, annual; and unpublished data).

ing 33% of all injury deaths caused by mechanical energy (U.S. Bureau of the Census, 1982; Baker, O'Neill & Karpf, 1984).

Christoffel vividly notes that the annual death toll in American MVAs is roughly equivalent to a *daily* airline tragedy involving 137 victims (1984). Recent evidence from the Department of Transportation, however, points to an optimistic trend (DOT, 1984). In the last three years a further reduction in traffic fatalities has been observed. In 1983, some 43,028 individuals perished in MVAs. This represents a 16% reduction from 1980, and a drop of 24% since 1972, when MVA fatalities were the highest in American history. At the same time, we should note that some groups are at greater risk of MVA death than others.

If we break down overall mortality into age and sex categories,

TABLE 2

Motor Vehicle Accidents -- Number and Deaths

1960 to 1980

	1960	1965	1970	1974	1975
Motor Vehicle Accidents (on and off road)[1]	11.4	14.7	22.1	23.7	24.9
Motor Vehicle Deaths Within 1 Year[2]	38.1	49.2	54.6	46.4	45.9
Traffic Death Rates [3]					
• per 100,000 resident population	20.2	24.3	25.8	21.2	20.7
• per 100,0000 registered vehicles	48.9	51.3	47.3	33.5	32.3
• per 100 million vehicle miles	5.1	5.3	4.7	3.5	3.4
• per 100,000 licensed drivers	41.7	47.8	47.2	36.0	34.3
Motor Vehicle Injuries[4]	3,078	3,982	4,983	4,634	4,978
Economic Loss[4,5]	10.2	14.2	23.5	30.4	36.1

[1] Expressed in millions of accidents; includes all motor vehicle accidents on and off the road and all injuries regardless of length of disability. Source: Insurance Information Institute, New York, *Insurance Facts*.

[2] Expressed in thousands of deaths; deaths that occur within one year of accident.

[3] Deaths within 30 days of accident. Source: U.S. National Highway Traffic Safety Administration, unpublished data.

TABLE 2

Motor Vehicle Accidents -- Number and Deaths

1960 to 1980

(continued)

	1976	1977	1978	1979	1980
Motor Vehicle Accidents (on and off road)[1]	25.4	26.7	27.7	26.7	24.1
Motor Vehicle Deaths Within 1 Year[2]	47.0	49.5	52.4	52.8	52.6
Traffic Death Rates [3]					
• per 100,000 resident population	20.9	21.8	22.7	22.8	22.6
• per 100,0000 registered vehicles	31.7	32.5	32.8	32.0	31.6
• per 100 million vehicle miles	3.3	3.3	3.3	3.3	3.3
• per 100,000 licensed drivers	34.0	34.7	35.7	35.7	35.2
Motor Vehicle Injuries[4]	5,269	5,575	5,798	5,681	5,230
Economic Loss[4,5]	40.9	46.5	52.6	56.4	57.1

[4] Expressed in thousands of injuries; includes all motor vehicle accidents on and off the road and all injuries regardless of length of disability. Source: Insurance Information Institute, New York, Insurance Facts.

[5] Expressed in billions of dollars; wage loss, legal, medical, hospital and funeral expenses, insurance and administrative costs, and property damage.

Source: Statistical Abstract of the United States, 1982-83, 1982, p.615.

the epidemic of motor vehicle accidents is self-evident. A disproportionate number of young males, primarily those in the teens and early twenties, are particularly vulnerable. Note that males have a 34% higher age-adjusted mortality rate than females (standardized to the United States general population in 1975). Overwhelmingly, the evidence indicates that the first four decades of life are especially precarious as far as accidental injury (MVA and other) is concerned, and the death and injury rates from MVAs for males 15-24 years of age are higher than for any other sex/age group (see Table 4) (Baker, O'Neill & Karpf, 1984; Dole, 1984; Fingerhut, Wilson & Feldman, 1980; Hartunian, Smart & Thompson, 1980; Nichols, 1982; Robertson, 1983a, 1983b; Trunkey, 1983a; U.S. Bureau of the Census, 1982; Warner, 1982; Will, 1977). To state this problem in graphic terms, "more than one in every 100 15-year-old boys will die in an accident before the age of 25, a death rate 20 times higher than that attributable to polio at its worst" (Warner, 1982, p. 7).

As in the case of other forms of morbidity and causes of death, race and socio-economic status are important variables in MVAs (cf. Syme & Berkman, 1981). Native Americans experience the highest fatality rates, followed by whites, blacks, and Asians (51, 24, 19, and 9 deaths per 100,000 respectively in the period 1977-1979) (Baker, O'Neill & Karpf, 1984). An inverse relationship exists between SES and MVA death rates, which has been

TABLE 3

Deaths from Motor Vehicle Accidents

1970 - 1979*

1970	54,845
1972	56,528
1975	46,032
1977	49,740
1978	52,653
1979	53,786

*Data differ from Table 2 because data are based on date of death rather than date of accident.

Source: Statistical Abstract of the United States, 1982-83, 1982, p. 616. (Based on U.S. NCHS Vital Statistics of the United States, annual; and unpublished data.)

TABLE 4

Incidence of Motor Vehicle Injuries
by Age and Sex, 1975

	Motor Vehicle Injuries*	Age-Specific Incidence Rates (per 100,000)
MALES		
0-14	275,520	10.1
15-24	997,434	49.0
25-34	492,651	32.1
35-44	229,600	20.6
45-54	185,693	16.2
55-64	127,720	13.7
65-74	73,346	12.2
> 75	34,188	10.9
Total Males	2,416,152	
FEMALES		
0-14	227,905	8.7
15-24	657,827	33.0
25-34	342,609	22.0
35-44	196,149	16.8
45-54	179,422	14.6
55-64	131,884	12.6
65-74	76,430	9.7
> 75	42,017	7.8
Total Females	1,854,243	
TOTAL POPULATION	4,270,395	

Age-Adjusted Motor Vehicle Injury Rates per 1,000 population (adjusted to U.S. General Population in 1975):
    Males = 22.92
    Females = 17.12
*Source: Hartunian et al., 1980:1253.

explained in terms of poorer quality roads, older vehicles, and lower quality medical care in low-income areas (Baker, O'Neill & Karpf, 1984; McKinlay, McKinlay, Jennings & Grant, 1983). Rural dwellers also have substantially higher death rates from MVAs (a ratio of 5 to 1) than do urban residents (Baker, O'Neill & Karpf, 1984).

In terms of the sheer numbers of people affected by MVAs in 1975, *fewer* people (in toto) were struck by cancer, coronary heart disease and stroke than were injured in MVAs (Hartunian, Smart & Thompson, 1980). When considering estimates of the costs of MVAs, the figures are quite striking. From Table 2, we see an increasingly larger economic loss (direct and indirect costs)[1] associated with MVAs, which reached a high of $57.1 billion in 1980. Based on elaborate economic calculations, Hartunian and associates (1980) estimate that only cancer supercedes MVA injuries in the costs incurred by individuals and society (cf. Grabow, Offord & Rieder, 1984).

To comprehend the sobering magnitude of MVA fatalities, it can be compared with other national tragedies. According to statistics from the U.S. Department of Defense, there were 33,629 battle deaths and 54,246 total deaths in the Korean war. In Vietnam, 47,269 service personnel perished in battle and an additional 10,670 names appear on the Vietnam Memorial in Washington, DC; i.e., soldiers believed to be dead or still missing-in-action (Karnow, 1983; U.S. Bureau of the Census, 1983). One can only speculate on the number of injuries (physical, psychological and social) sustained by American soldiers and other military personnel in these wars. It should be noted further that the average age of the American soldier in Vietnam was 19 years (Karnow, 1983). *Each* year almost as many Americans are killed in MVAs as died in each of these two wars, which are regarded as national tragedies. Many of those afflicted are no older than the soldiers who fought in Vietnam. "Trauma," a term customarily reserved to describe the consequences of war, is now a major killer in America at peace. Yet despite the gravity of the situation, comparatively little is being done to curb it.

BACKGROUND CONCEPTS

While the epidemic of injury and death from MVAs demands high priority and a coherent and adequate policy response, none is as yet forthcoming. *Prevention* is clearly the key to reducing the scope of this tragedy. Before exploring some specific policy options with respect to MVA injury and death, we introduce two concepts which will provide a framework for the ensuing discussion. These are, respectively, "refocusing upstream" (from the political economy of illness) and "appropriate technology" (from the study of health in the developing world).

Refocusing Upstream

Within the last decade, considerable attention (Green, 1984; Haggerty, 1977; Hamburg, Elliott & Parron, 1982; Leichter, 1981) has been focused on personal lifestyles and environmental determinants of health and illness. For example, the report *A New Perspective on the Health of Canadians* issued by former Canadian Minister of Health and Welfare Marc Lalonde (1974) suggested that much ill-health and premature death could be prevented through modification of at-risk behaviors (e.g., proper dietary intake, regular exercise, smoking cessation, etc.). Other reports in this vein were published in the United States (U.S. Department of Health, Education & Welfare, 1979) and in Great Britain (*Prevention and Health: Everybody's Business*, 1976) which challenged the parochialism of the biomedical model of disease, while embracing a more holistic perspective of the causes, correlates and solutions of premature mortality and increased morbidity. As infectious diseases have been replaced by chronic diseases, and since 50% of mortality from the 10 leading causes of death can be traced to lifestyle (Hamburg, Elliott & Parron, 1982), it is clearly on this front that strategic efforts should be focused.

John Knowles argued that the responsibility for health clearly lies with the individual (1981). Although Knowles' indictment of personal living styles has merit, when taken to its logical extreme, it absolves the "manufacturers of illness" of their responsibilities. ("Manufacturers of illness" are those individuals, interest groups and organizations, which, in addition to providing material goods and services, also produce, as an inevitable byproduct, widespread morbidity and mortality [McKinlay, 1981a]). Knowles' decontextualization of many health problems and moralistic tone exemplify a "victim-blaming ideology" which is incapable of understanding the essence of major health problems and instead shifts the burden of responsibility to the individual (Crawford, 1981; Labonte, 1983). The solutions to the most urgent health problems obviously require preventive measures and a critical examination of the pathogenic nature of our political economy if interventions are ever to ameliorate these problems.

The current emphasis on personal culpability for at-risk behavior has been successfully propagated by the manufacturers of illness (McKinlay, 1978, 1981a). By interweaving at-risk behaviors with the dominant cultural value system, artificial needs are easily manufactured. Failure to conform with these cultural imperatives is little short of rejection of that which is near and dear to society's members. The point at which the organized health care system generally enters is *downstream*, where there is "evidence" of individuals' failures to live up to artificially contrived norms. Interventions at this point, while necessary, tend to offer little more than palliation (for chronic conditions) but are characterized by progressive beneficence on the part of the manufacturers of illness. Were there a more critical appreciation of the origins of illness (Eyer, 1984), interventions would occur *upstream* through regulation of the political-economic institutions clearly culpable for morbidity and mortality in the first place.

Numerous examples exist of the actions of the manufacturers of illness (cf. Navarro, 1976; Waitzkin, 1983, 1983b). The case of the food industry has been extensively explored (McKinlay, 1981a). Automobile usage provides a further illustration of the "downstream" endeavors prevalent in American society. As noted by Warner (1982, 1983), the automobile is the quintessential symbol of American affluence and progress and the American people's love affair with the automobile has been unwavering ever since Ford rolled the first Model T off the assembly line. Buying a car, or using one's parents' car, is a rite of passage for Western youth. The car has been inextricably bound with youth and coming of age. The popular culture has also enshrined the automobile, e.g., in television ("Route 66" and "Night Rider"), films (e.g., "Bullit," "The Love Bug" and the "Smokey and the Bandit" trilogy), and songs (the Beach Boys' musical anthology about cars included "Little GTO," "Little Ol' Lady from Pasadena," "Fun, Fun, Fun," the Beatles' "Drive My Car," "Radar Love" and Janis Joplin's "Lord, Won't Ya Buy Me A Mercedes-Benz?").

Ever responsive to the perceived "needs" of the public, automobile manufacturers have designed the "ultimate driving machine" (the commercial slogan for BMW). Cars today can be equipped with every imaginable option, including internal mechanisms which "speak" through a computerized, synthesized voice to passengers. Manufacturers have gone out of their way to market a product the consumer cannot resist. Recall Toyota's marketing slogan "You asked for it . . . You got it . . . Toyota," or General

Motor's question "Wouldn't you really rather drive a Buick?" Sometimes in their zeal to get their product on the market, however, tragic compromises in designs have been made, as exemplified in the Ford Pinto's tendency to ignite on impact.

Over time, in response to humanistic concerns expressed by consumer advocates such as Ralph Nader (1965), car companies have had to incorporate safety mechanisms into the design of automobiles; these consist mostly of crash worthiness and crash avoidance features. In 1966, under the Johnson administration, the Department of Transportation ordered car manufacturers to install manual safety belts in new cars, effective in the 1968 model year. A vigorous debate on restraining devices in motor vehicles has raged ever since, most recently fueled by the proclamation by U.S. Secretary of Transportation (Elizabeth Dole) that by the model year 1989, 100% of all automobiles manufactured for the U.S. market must have automatic occupant restraints (i.e., air bags which inflate upon impact or automatic seat belts which wrap around passengers as they close car doors).[2]

Some years ago, Senator Moynihan of New York wrote that the automobile is "a prime agent of risk-taking in a society that still values risk-taking, but does not provide many outlets" (quoted in Will, 1977). Indeed, the driving habits of Americans are a major factor contributing to premature death and chronic disability. Instead of willingly equipping automobiles with features which lessen drivers' (and passengers' and pedestrians') vulnerabilities, car manufacturers have been consistently obstinate, undertaking changes only when forced to do so. The arguments by motor vehicle companies which challenge the efficacy and cost-effectiveness of safety features, such as air bags, are largely specious. The auto manufacturers are not alone in this resistance; in their company there is the insurance industry and those health care institutions set up to put people together again once the damage has been done (e.g., trauma and emergency medical centers, rehabilitative technicians and therapists). An entire substructure has been built up to handle the current epidemic of MVAs. Many lives have been saved by emergency medical technicians; no one can question the necessity for such downstream endeavors. The problem remains, however, that the current set of interventions (trauma centers which come too late and appeals to the public to "buckle up" for safety) remind one of "the ambulance at the bottom of the cliff." Health institutions continue to attribute responsibility to the individual, instead of insisting that manufacturers make the safest possible car and that legislators insure optimally danger-free road conditions. These approaches fail to take into account the social contexts that reinforce the very behaviors which must be changed.

Appropriate Technology

Under the leadership of Director-General Halfdan Mahler, the World Health Organization (WHO) has adopted the goal of "health for all by the year 2000." Considering that most of the world's population has limited or no access to essential medical and health services and that the majority of deaths and causes of illness and disability are preventable, this optimistic declaration was intended as a manifesto for meeting health challenges in developing societies. We argue that developed societies might also benefit from this political and organizational strategy.

At the International Conference on Primary Health Care in Alma Ata in 1978, the cornerstone of the policy for achieving "health for all" included the following: the deployment of *appropriate technology* (i.e., technology which has proven efficacy, is culturally and socially acceptable and economically feasible for those adopting it), a primary care system operating on the basis of a *multisectoral approach* (i.e., one informed by the knowledge that social, political and economic factors affect the health of populations as much as if not more than the health sector, per se) and finally, the mandate for *community involvement*. At the heart of the primary health care approach is a call for the demonstration of effectiveness and efficiency (Cochrane, 1972; McKinlay, 1979) in interventions designed to enhance the health of populations. In addition, it requires individuals to exercise some autonomous control over the factors affecting their lives and health (Illich, 1973).

Of course, the problems of developing countries are, in many important respects, different from those confronting the West. The major causes of death in the Third and Fourth worlds are of an infectious nature; diarrheal and intestinal parasitic diseases account for a sizeable proportion of premature death and disability. Poverty and malnutrition are the primary contributing factors in lowered life expectancy throughout much of the developing world. To deal with these kind of problems requires political will and the rational allocation of resources.

Also essential is the deployment of appropriate technology,

including appropriate levels of manpower skill (Acuna, 1980; Browne, 1980). For example, programs assuring clean sources of water and appropriate waste disposal would do much to reduce mortality and disabling morbidity (Grant, 1983; Morley, Rohde & Williams, 1983). Similarly, in areas where malaria is endemic, the use of pesticides has been both an effective and appropriate intervention (Golladay, 1980). Maternal and child health programs (including prenatal and well-baby care, as well as skilled birth attendance) have significantly reduced infant morality rates in countries like India (Chand & Soni, 1983).

Because the health problems of the developing world are largely socio-economic, intervention programs must be tailored accordingly. However, the Western influence has fostered a desire for "magic bullets" and machines—solutions which are costly, not necessarily of demonstrated effectiveness, and inaccessible to large segments of society in the West as well as in developing countries (McKinlay, 1981). Bringing in coronary care units and specialist physicians is not the solution for the ills of the developing world. Instead, appropriate technology, suited to the epidemiologic, economic and socio-cultural characteristics of a society, is mandated. Pragmatically, preventive health programs throughout the life cycle are indispensable to achieving the WHO goal of "health for all."

The application of the concept of appropriate technology to a problem of development (MVA injury and death) rather than of underdevelopment may seem unclear, but its relevance is obvious. Any technology is appropriate if *it beneficially alters the natural course of disease or solves a health problem*; if *it is relevant and amenable to prevailing social conditions and available resources*; if *it is a cost efficient response* to a significant problem; and if *it increases access to effective health care*. Finally, a technology is appropriate if, while having all of the above features, *it also empowers individuals* ("the people's health in the people's hands").

Seat belts and air bags are clearly examples of appropriate technologies. As many studies have shown, these forms of restraint save lives and prevent injury. They are effective, cost-efficient, and ultimately enhance the quality of individuals' lives, if for no other reason than that they act as mediators between two fragile entities—one human, one technological. If seat belts and air bags are "appropriate" and further, constitute an "upstream" response to the issue of auto safety, why then has there been such resistance to their use? One answer to this query is given by J. N. Morris:

The main issue must therefore be over what the government should be doing, and this is mixed up in philosophic and political dilemmas concerning the liberty of the individual versus the claims of the common good, and the disadvantages of paternalism against the responsibilities of the community. Meanwhile, ruthless commercial interests usually manage to keep a step or two ahead and altogether too little is done to enable people to mend their ways (1982, p. 11).

AVAILABLE POLICY OPTIONS FOR MOTOR VEHICLE ACCIDENT MORTALITY AND INJURY

According to conservative estimates, in excess of 40,000 individuals will lose their lives on American roads this year alone. Fifty times that many will experience an injury while an occupant of a motor vehicle. Given what is known of the hazards of driving, what measures have been taken to lessen this toll?

First, since 1966, the Department of Transportation (through such agencies as the National Highway Traffic Safety Administration) has been regulating the automobile industry to ensure car crash worthiness and crash avoidance capabilities (e.g., through shatter-proof glass, padded dashboards, hydraulic brake systems, energy-absorbing steering wheel columns, and manual lap/shoulder seat belts). According to Robertson (1981), in the period between 1975 and 1978, had these safety regulations not been in effect some 37,000 more people would have perished in MVAs than the already alarming 194,800.

Second, the strict enforcement of the "55 Saves Lives" campaign (the Federal government threatened loss of Federal highway dollars to states failing to enforce the speed limit) with resultant narrowing of speed distributions resulted in lower accident and mortality rates. According to a report in the *New York Times*, (Fifty-five mph, 1983) some 45,000 lives have been spared since the enactment of the federal speed limit *ten years ago*. Far from inconsequential was the energy crisis of the mid-70s which contributed to the decline in MVA mortality (Warner, 1982; 1983), as fewer people took to the roads. The 55 mph speed limit has in fact been a significant public policy. Legislators did not envision the positive, unanticipated public health consequences of the speed limit, which was implemented in response to the national energy shortage caused by a quadrupling of oil prices by the Arab cartel.

A very significant defense against MVA injury and death is usage of one of three types of restraint systems: manual lap/shoulder safety belts, automatic safety belts, and air bags which inflate upon impact. While all cars on the American market are now equipped with manual belts, only 12%[3] of the driving public *correctly* uses these safety devices, according to the NHTSA (Henderson, 1984a, 1984b; Nichols, 1982). A recent Gallup poll (1984) found that 25% of its sample reported using their seat belts the last time they were in the car, an 8 percentage point increase since 1982 (*Did you know*, 1984). It is hypothesized that if everyone buckled up, traffic fatalities could be cut in half. The reasons for failure to use manual belts have been related to inconvenience, discomfort, and fears of entrapment (Insurance Institute for Highway Safety, 1983; Nichols, 1982; Warner, 1982, 1983). Researchers also note that nonuse results from insensitive perceptions of the probability of being involved in a serious MVA (1 chance in 100 over the driving lifetime of being involved in a fatal accident; 1 chance in 3 of at least one disabling injury), and individuals' gross underestimation of their risks of involvement in an MVA (Robertson, 1976, 1977; 1983a; Warner, 1982, 1983).

Because few people voluntarily use seat belts, despite their proven effectiveness, coercive legislation has been required to ensure that all drivers, and their passengers, use seat belts under threat of fines. Such mandatory laws are in effect in more than 40 states, countries, or provinces (Nichols, 1982; Transport Canada, 1982). The pioneer country was Australia in 1970, and one of the most recent U.S. additions is New York State, where a law became effective January 1, 1985 (Charlton, 1984; Goodwin, 1984; Molotsky, 1984; Simmons, 1984).[4]

There is no doubt as to the efficacy of seat belts in reducing injuries and deaths in MVAs. Table 5 summarizes the experiences in four sites (cf. O'Neill, 1982, p. 105). National data for Canada (in which only the provinces of Alberta and Prince Edward Island are without mandatory seat belt legislation) show an overall reduction in deaths and injury in excess of 17% for 1983, compared with the previous year (Gruson, 1984). Since the 1981 enactment of seat belt laws in Great Britain, estimates are that 95% of drivers and front seat passengers comply with the law, and fatal and serious injuries have been reduced by 25%. Within 8 months of its passage, British

TABLE 5

Summary of Seat Belt Law Effectiveness Around the World

	AUSTRALIA	FRANCE	BELGIUM	ONTARIO, CANADA
Date of Law	Jan. 1972	July 1973	June 1975	Jan. 1976
Penalty	$20 (max.)	$20 (max.)	$15 (max.)	$100 (max.)
Enforcement	yes	yes	yes	yes
Public Information Program	yes	yes	yes	yes
Pre-Law Usage	25%	26%	17%	17%
Post-Law Usage	68-85%	64-85%	92%	64-77%
Injury Reduction*	20%	32%	24%	15%
Fatality Reduction*	25%	22%	39%	17%

Source: Nichols, 1982:65 (based on research reports by Ziegler, 1977 and DOT, 1980).

*It is noteworthy that even mandating seat belt use does not fully solve the problem of MVA injury and fatality, suggesting that such laws are not enough and should be complemented by other preventive and regulatory measures.

observers claim that 350 lives were saved and 4,500 serious injuries prevented as a result of this law (Avery, 1984). Its success has prompted legislators to consider seriously a law requiring backseat passengers to buckle up as well (Avery, 1984).

Despite these successes in numerous jurisdictions, there has been vociferous opposition to such laws in the United States. A recent Gallup poll showed that 65% of the population oppose such legislation, compared to 30% favoring it (*Did you know*, 1984). Seen as yet another example of state intrusion into the private affairs of citizens, such laws have been called coercive and paternalistic

(Courtwright, 1980; Noble, 1984; Wikler, 1978). These charges notwithstanding, the inevitability of such laws seems apparent, especially in the light of Secretary Dole's reinstatement of Federal Motor Vehicle Safety Standard 208. Automobile manufacturers now enthusiastically support mandatory seat belt laws and have openly acknowledged that they will lobby hard to avoid having to install passive restraints (Henderson, 1984a, 1984b; Barron, 1984; Slouching, 1984; *Playing safe*, 1984).

Because of the public's disinclination toward legislated or voluntary buckling up, many have suggested passive restraints as an alternative which is not so dependent on the whims of individuals. The two most widely cited passive restraints (air bags and automatic seat belts) both provide demonstrable benefits, but each carries special problems. Automatic seat belts are easily detachable, and thus their effectiveness is dubious. In this event, as Warner notes, "the individual converts the passive restraint system into an active nonrestraint system, and effectiveness goes to zero" (1982, p. 23).

Air bags, on the other hand, are supported as an effective, albeit more costly, technology for the prevention of MVA death and injury (Christoffel, 1984; Insurance Information Institute, 1984; Karr, 1976; Passel, 1983; Warner, 1982, 1983) and have the important advantage over automatic or manual seat belts in that they are used when needed and are effectively independent of human volition or action (Warner, 1982). Within 1/100th of a second after a 12 mph impact, the bag inflates, acting as a barrier between the driver and the windshield. It is estimated that more than 12,000 lives could be saved and 100,000 critical injuries prevented if air bags were a standard feature in all cars on the U.S. market (Warner, 1982). Effectiveness aside, GM claims that consumers are unwilling to pay for this option (Christoffel, 1984; Karr, 1976). A 1984 Gallup poll found, however, that 60% favored a law requiring mandatory air bags (*Did you know*, 1984).

While air bags are obviously not foolproof, when used in conjunction with seat belts, the savings in lives (and costs of injury and death) is thought to be formidable.[5] At present, however, industry analysts see the issue as an "either/or" one—either mandatory seat belt legislation or passive restraints; either automatic seat belts or air bags. Contrarily, these restraining devices should be viewed as adjuncts to one another (Warner, 1982; Christoffel, 1984) if, indeed, the objective is "to select a national protection strategy which offers the greatest potential for saving lives and reducing suffering" (DOT, 1984). Although Secretary Dole's reinstatement of Federal Motor Vehicle Safety Standard (FMVSS) 208 would have all cars equipped with passive restraints by 1989, it should be noted that:

— The "Big Three" auto manufacturers (GM, Ford, and Chrysler) have begun an active campaign hoping that states will voluntarily implement mandatory seat belt laws.
— Simultaneously, all three are concentrating on improving the crash-worthiness of automobiles, since FMVSS 208 would be ineffectual if cars could be shown to protect unrestrained passengers in a 30 mph crash (Barron, 1984a; 1984b).
— Air bags have been installed in more than 10,000 cars since 1972 (mostly in large-size and luxury models). Whether one can generalize from this experience to all other models is in doubt. Of equal importance is the fact that, until now, access to passive restraints has been unequal. If FMVSS 208 is fully implemented it will not be until 1989 that everyone behind the wheel will have full access to passive restraints. And this eventuality is hardly guaranteed.

A third option exists for dealing with MVA injury and death: acute, emergency medical and surgical (EMS) care (trauma centers). Strongly influenced by military medical corps triage procedures, today's trauma center is designed to deal expeditiously with a vast array of critical injuries, not the least of which include those from MVAs (estimated to constitute 15% of all hospital admissions and close to 32% of the deaths caused by external trauma) (Barancik, Chatterjee, Greene, Michenzi & Fife, 1983; Nickerson, 1984). Like the MASH units in Korea and Vietnam, the underlying principle of EMS care is to take the injured immediately to a source of definitive care, where the necessary manpower and facilities are available.

How does a trauma center differ from regular emergency room care? Solely concerned with trauma patients, it is a facility providing 24-hour "in house" emergency and medical services. Unlike standard emergency room facilities, the medical staff includes trauma surgeons, anesthesiologists, physicians trained in emergency room care and several subspecialists (e.g., neurosurgeons, thoracic surgeons, orthopedists, urologists, radiologists, internists and pediatricians). In addition, support staff includes a cadre of highly trained nurses and ancillary technicians (Jarriel,

1980; Nickerson, 1984; Pacer, 1983; Trunkey, 1983a; Williams, 1983). Availability on a full-time basis of a fully-staffed operating room, a blood bank and other back-up medical services is vital to the effectiveness of EMS units. Although trauma care was not initially embraced with enthusiasm, events such as the assassination attempt on President Reagan and the speed with which his gunshot wounds were taken care of spurred interest in the concept of EMS systems. Other countries (e.g., Germany) have also shown increased interest in trauma facilities (Trunkey, 1983a, 1983b).

According to the American College of Surgeons Committee on Trauma, which has endorsed and established guidelines for such facilities, the cost of EMS units is substantial. Based on 1977 estimates of minimum staffing requirements and the necessary in house infrastructure, the optimal EMS unit would cost in excess of $3.6 million annually; this figure does not include several of the key back-up personnel (Teuful & Trunkey, 1977). In order to constitute an effective and cost-efficient unit, it is estimated that between 400 and 1,000 (depending on the level of the EMS unit) victims of traumatic injuries would need to be seen per year in each unit (Eggold, 1983).

Trauma experts estimate that as many as 30% of those who die from serious injuries (e.g., central nervous system injuries, multiple fractures, gunshot wounds, etc.) could be saved if dispatched quickly to an EMS facility (Nickerson, 1984). However, the evidence for the effectiveness of such units by type of trauma is only beginning to be known. In a review of traumatic injuries (MVA and other) treated in Orange County, California, West and associates (1983) report that critically wounded persons' survival is greatly enhanced if treated in an EMS unit. Of 39 patients treated in a trauma center, 5% died of a potentially preventable death, compared with 72% of the 57 patients treated at existing, nontrauma facilities. Trunkey's research in San Francisco supports this conclusion (1983b). A study comparing trauma victims taken to two sites (one with a trauma unit and the other without) showed that those cared for in the trauma unit had substantially higher survival rates and fewer preventable deaths (West, Trunkey & Lim, 1979). Available evidence supports the conclusion that severely injured persons are at a marked disadvantage if taken to a hospital without a trauma facility (Trunkey, 1983a, 1983b).

It would be easy to embrace the concept of the trauma unit as a viable solution to critical injuries such as those sustained in MVAs, on the assumption that this type of socialized facility could better manage trauma. Despite a lacuna in the research evidence, trauma units have proliferated throughout America in recent years (Jarriel, 1980), a situation not unlike that of coronary care units (Waitzkin, 1983a, 1983b). Indeed, the parallels between CCUs and trauma units are striking. Both are extremely expensive as capital- and labor-intensive interventions. Consideration of the governmental and commercial motivations in the burgeoning of trauma centers is, however, beyond the scope of this paper.

It has been noted that "trauma slices socio-economic barriers" (Pacer, 1983, p. 30). A significant question remains: do trauma centers provide adequate access to emergency services, independent of socioeconomic criteria? In other words, efficacy and fiscal considerations aside, do all socioeconomic groups have equal access to trauma centers? The answer is probably no. Rural areas have fewer EMS and general hospital facilities (Conn, 1983). The negative experience of low income and minority populations in standard emergency rooms (e.g., Himmelstein, Woolhandler, Harnly, Bader, Silber, Backer & Jones, 1984; Roth, 1972; Sudnow, 1978) is probably pertinent here.

While Trunkey has noted that "the U.S. can no longer afford the present rate of preventable death and disability resulting from trauma" and that "the search for solutions to the trauma problem must become a national priority" (1983a, p. 35), we remain unconvinced that, in terms of efficacy, cost effectiveness, social acceptability and accessibility, the trauma center is the best means for handling the epidemic of critical injuries sustained in MVAs in the United States. This "downstream" endeavor only provides a post hoc solution to the problem of trauma, without getting to the structural origins of the problem. "Upstream" approaches, on the other hand, including mandatory seat belt legislation, regulation of the automobile industry to install passive restraints, and intensive public education programs as preventive strategies, have been shown to reduce considerably the potential mortality and morbidity associated with driving in America. The "appropriateness" of these interventions is beyond dispute.

CONCLUSION

Haddon (1980, p. 418), one of the foremost experts in injury epidemiology, has suggested ten strategies to counter the rising tide of injuries sustained in America. These are:

1. to prevent the creation of the hazard in the first place;
2. to reduce the amount of hazard brought into being;
3. to prevent the release of the hazard that already exists;
4. to modify the rate or spatial distribution of release of the hazard from its source;
5. to separate, in time or space, the hazard and that which is to be protected;
6. to separate the hazard and that which is to be protected by interposition of a material barrier;
7. to modify relevant basic qualities of the hazard;
8. to make what is to be protected more resistant to damage from the hazard;
9. to begin to counter the damage already done by the environmental hazard; and
10. to stabilize, repair and rehabilitate the object of the damage.

Applied to the problem of MVA injuries, a wide range of interventions (not only those calling for improvements in drivers' behavior) is suggested (Robertson, 1983b). Interventions which misplace responsibility for the problem of MVA injury and death by focusing on individuals only will fail to resolve this problem. Changes in individual behavior (e.g., more prudent driving habits and the usage of internal car restraints) will substantially lessen the tragedy of MVAs. But changes to vehicles and road conditions (interventions with a political-economic and preventive focus) will have a much more formidable impact on the annual motor vehicle casualty rate.

NOTES

1. Direct and indirect costs include the following: wage loss, legal and medical expenses, insurance administration costs and property damage. Other incidental expenses (e.g., the cost absorbed by public agencies such as the police and fire departments) are not included in these estimates.

2. This edict has an all-important loophole however. If states containing two-thirds of the U.S. population enact mandatory seat belt legislation, the passive restraint requirement (Federal Motor Vehicle Safety Standard 208) will be rescinded.

3. One should note the following frequently cited correlates of seat belt usage: higher education, highway driving, perceived health concern, urban (within SMSA) residence, females, drivers of small vehicles, those who have taken driver education courses, drivers of new cars, those with comfortable or convenient belt systems and lastly, those residing and driving in the western U.S. (Nichols, 1982; Warner, 1982; 1983).

4. Child passenger safety legislation has been enacted in all states except Texas and Wyoming, where laws are pending (DOT, 1984). In the short period between 1981-1983, such laws contributed to a 10% reduction in death to children aged 0-4 involved in MVAs. DOT estimates that as of 1983, 60% of all infants and 38% of all toddlers are being restrained in safety seats when passengers in cars (for further information on child restraint programs see Ershoff & Wasserman, 1982; Meyer, 1981; Page, 1984; Williams, 1979, 1983; Williams, Karpf & Zador, 1983; Williams & Wells, 1981). In a less optimistic vein, deaths on motorcycles have risen sharply since 1976, when 27 states repealed helmet laws (Baker & Teret, 1981). Motorcycle deaths account for 1/10 of all traffic deaths. Like seat belt restraints, helmet laws have been hotly debated (e.g., Baker & Teret, 1981; Perkins, 1981; Watson, Zador & Wilks, 1981) with the central concern being the presumed paternalistic nature of such laws (Courtwright, 1980; Wikler, 1978; Yankauer, 1981).

5. Cost-benefit analyses indicate that the net savings could amount to between $3.4 and $8.5 billion (1981 dollars) after passive seat belts are universal. The net benefit of air bags is estimated to be in the neighborhood of $4.9–$6.6 billion (1981 dollars) (Arnould Grabowski, 1981, cited in Warner, 1982). Nordhaus (1981) calculates that complete rescission of FMVSS 208 will amount to $69 billion in net social costs. He has noted:

> The passive restraint rule is, from an economic point of view, as important as any environmental, health, or safety rule on the books. If the estimates of the impact on fatalities are accurate, a rescission would be equivalent to repealing a law that cuts in half the homicide rate. It is equivalent to forgoing the medical advances that allowed the virtual elimination of death from tuberculosis over the last quarter century (in Warner, 1982, p. 32).

REFERENCES

Acuna, H. R. (1980). Appropriate technology for health. *Bulletin of the Pan American Health Organization, 14*, 221-223.

Avery, J. G. (1984). Seat belt success: Where next? *British Medical Journal, 288*, 662-663.

Baker, S. P., O'Neill, B. & Karpf, R. S. (1984). *The Injury Fact Book*. Lexington: Lexington Books.

Baker, S. & Teret, S. (1981). Freedom and protection: A balancing of interests. *American Journal of Public Health, 71*, 295-297.

Barancik, J. I., Chatterjee, B. F., Greene, Y. C., Michenzi, E. M. & Fife, D. (1983). Northeastern Ohio trauma study: I. Magnitude of the problem. *American Journal of Public Health, 73*, 746-751.

Barron, J. (1984a, July 12). Auto makers hoping state laws save them from air bags ruling. *New York Times*.

Barron, J. (1984b, July 13). Detroit expects problems from air bag decision. *New York Times*.

Browne, S. G. (1980). Appropriate technologies for the future. *Royal Society of London Bulletin, 209*, 183-186.

Chand, A. D. & Soni, M. I. (1983). Evaluation in primary health care: A case study in India. In D. Morley, J. Rohde & G. Williams (eds.), *Practicing Health for All*. Oxford: Oxford University Press.

Charlton, T. (1984, June 26). New York approves law: Buck up or pay up. *Boston Globe*.

Christoffel, T. (1984). The supreme court and airbags. *American Journal of Public Health,* *74*, 269-270.

Cochrane, A. L. (1972). *Effectiveness and efficiency.* London: Nuffield Hospitals Trust.

Conn, A. (1983). Urban systems of trauma care: The Baltimore experience. In J. G. West, A. B. Gazzaniga & R. H. Cales (eds.), *Trauma care systems.* New York: Praeger.

Courtwright, D. T. (1980). Public health and public wealth: Social costs as a basis for restrictive policies. *Milbank Memorial Fund Quarterly/Health and Society, 58,* 268-282.

Crawford, R. (1977). You are dangerous to your health: The ideology and politics of victim-blaming. *International Journal of Health Service, 7,* 663-680.

Did you know? Seat belts and passive restraints. (1984, August). *Nations Health.*

DOT: Traffic deaths drop to 20-year low: 43,028. (1984, March). *Nations Health.*

Dole, E. H. (1984, July 11). *Secretary of Transportation: News Conference on Automatic Crash Protection,* Washington, DC.

Douglas, M. & Wildavsky, A. (1982). *Risk and culture: An essay on the selection of technical and environmental dangers.* Berkeley, CA: University of California Press.

Eggold, R. (1983). Trauma care regionalization: A necessity. *Journal of Trauma, 23,* 260-262.

Epstein, S. (1978). *The politics of cancer.* San Francisco: Sierra Club Books.

Ershoff, D. & Wasserman, F. (1982). Does health education provide a good return on investment? One HMO's experience with an infant car safety program. *The Group Health Journal, Summer,* 4-14.

Eyer, J. Capitalism, health and illness. In J. B. McKinlay (ed.), *Issues in the political economy of health care.* London: Tavistock.

Fifty-five mph speed limit said to have saved 45,000 lives. (1983, December 3). *New York Times.*

Fingerhut, L. A., Wilson, R. W. & Feldman, J. J. (1980). Health and disease in the United States. *Annual Review of Public Health, 1,* 1-36.

Friedman, G. D. (1980). *Primer of epidemiology* (2nd ed.). New York: McGraw-Hill Book Co.

Golladay, F. (1980). *Health-sector policy paper.* Washington, DC: World Bank.

Goodwin, M. (1984, July 13). Cuomo signs seat belt law and cites studies on safety. *New York Times.*

Grabow, J. D., Offord, K. P. & Rieder, M. E. (1984). The cost of head trauma in Olmsted County, Minnesota, 1970-74. *American Journal of Public Health, 74,* 710-717.

Grant, K. R. (1983). *From 'The technological imperative' to 'Appropriate technology': The challenge of health in the developing world.* Paper presented at the Eighth International Conference on the Social Sciences and Medicine, University of Stirling, Stirling, Scotland.

Green, L. W. (1984). Modifying and developing health behavior. *Annual Review of Public Health, 5,* 215-236.

Gruson, L. (1984, July 13). Ontario's seat belt law hailed for saving lives. *New York Times.*

Haddon, W. (1980). Advances in the epidemiology of injuries as a basis for public policy. *Public Health Reports, 95,* 411-421.

Haggerty, R. J. (1977). Changing lifestyles to improve health. *Preventive Medicine, 6,* 276-289.

Hamburg, D. A., Elliott, G. R. & Parron, D. L. (eds.) (1982). *Health and behavior: Frontiers of research in the behavioral sciences.* Washington, DC: National Academy Press.

Hartunian, N., Smart, C. & Thompson, M. (1980). The incidence and economic costs of cancer, motor vehicle injuries, coronary heart disease and stroke: A comparative analysis. *American Journal of Public Health, 70,* 1249-1260.

Henderson, N. (1984a, July 11). Seat belt law option expected. *Washington Post.*

Henderson, N. (1984b, July 12). U.S. presses seat belt laws. *Washington Post.*

Himmelstein, D. U., Woolhandler, S., Harnly, M., Bader, M. B., Silber, R., Backer, H. D.

& Jones, A. A. (1984). Patient transfers: Medical practice as social triage. *American Journal of Public Health, 74,* 494-497.

Illich, I. (1973). *Tools for conviviality.* New York: Harper and Row.

Insurance Information Institute. (1984). *Air bags: A matter of life or death.* New York: Insurance Information Institute.

Insurance Institute for Highway Safety. (1983, December 19). *The highway loss reduction status report.*

Jarriel, T. (1980, April 24). To save a life (20/20 news report). ABC News media transcript.

Karnow, S. (1983). *Vietnam: A history.* New York: Viking Press.

Karr, A. R. (1976, November 11). Saga of the air bag, or the slow deflation of a car safety idea. *Wall Street Journal.*

Knowles, J. H. The responsibility of the individual. In P. Conrad & R. Kern (eds.), *The sociology of health and illness.* New York: St. Martins Press.

Labonte, R. (1983). Good health: Individual or social. *Canadian Forum,* pp. 10-13.

Lalonde, M. (1974). *A new perspective on the health of Canadians.* Ottawa: Minister of Supply and Services.

Last, J. M. (1983). *A dictionary of epidemiology.* New York: Oxford University Press.

Leichter, H. (1981, October). Public policy and the British experience. *The Hastings Center Report,* pp. 32-39.

MacMahon, B. & Pugh, T. F. (1970). *Epidemiology: Principles and methods.* Boston: Little, Brown and Co.

McKinlay, J. B. (1978). On the medical-industrial complex. *Monthly Review, 30,* 38-42.

McKinlay, J. B. (1979). Epidemiological and political determinants of social policies regarding the public health. *Social Science Medicine, 13,* 541-558.

McKinlay, J. B. (1981a). A case for refocussing upstream: The political economy of illness. In P. Conrad & R. Kerns (eds.), *Sociology of health and illness: Critical perspectives.* New York: St. Martins Press.

McKinlay, J. B. (1981b). From 'Promising report' to 'Standard procedure': Seven stages in the career of a medical innovation. *Milbank Memorial Fund Quarterly/Health and Society, 59,* 376-411.

McKinlay, J. B., McKinlay, S. M., Jennings, S. E. & Grant, K. R. (1983). Mortality, morbidity and the inverse care law. In A. L. Greer & S. Greer (eds.), *Cities and sickness: Health care in urban America.* Beverly Hills, CA: Sage.

Meyer, R. J. (1981). Save the child: Children and automobile restraints. *American Journal of Public Health, 71,* 122-123.

Molotsky, I. (1984, July 12). U.S. sets '89 date for car air bags but gives choice. *New York Times.*

Morley, D., Rohde, J. & Williams, G. (eds.) (1983). *Practicing health for all.* Oxford: Oxford University Press.

Morris, J. N. (1982). Epidemiology and prevention. *Milbank Memorial Fund Quarterly/Health and Society, 60,* 1-16.

Nader, R. (1965). *Unsafe at any speed.* New York: Grossman.

National Highway Traffic Safety Administration Traffic Safety Programs. (1980). *Child restraints: Issue paper.* Washington, DC: U.S. Dept. of Transportation, DOT HS-803 819.

Navarro, V. (1976). *Medicine under capitalism.* New York: Prodist.

Nichols, J. L. (1982). *Effectiveness and efficiency of safety belt and child restraint usage programs.* Washington, DC: U.S. Dept. of Transportation, National Highway Traffic Safety Administration, NHTSA Technical Report, DOT HS-806 142.

Nickerson, C. (1984, February 20). Trauma. *Boston Globe,* pp. 37-38.

Noble, K. B. (1984, July 15). The politics of safety has a life of its own. *New York Times.*

O'Neill, P. D. (1982). *Health crisis 2000.* Copenhagen: World Health Organization.

Pacer, W. P. (1983). *Trauma centers: Decertification and dedesignation.* Paper presented at the 111th annual Meeting of the American Public Health Association, Dallas, TX.

Page, R. M. (1982). *Relationships among parental seat belt intentions and attitudinal factors concerning child car seats*. Unpublished manuscript.

Passel, P. (1983, December 18). What's holding back air bags? *New York Times Magazine*.

Perkins, R. J. (1981). Perspective on the public good. *American Journal of Public Health, 71*, 294-295.

Playing safe on auto safety. (1984, July 13). *New York Times*.

Prevention and health: Everybody's business, a consultative document. (1976). London: HMSO.

Primary health care. (1978). Report of the International Conference on Primary Health Care, Alma Ata, USSR. Jointly sponsored by the World Health Organization and the United Nations Children's Fund. Geneva: World Health Organization.

Robertson, L. S. (1976). Estimates of motor vehicle seat belt effectiveness and use: Implications for occupant crash protection. *American Journal of Public Health, 66*, 859-864.

Robertson, L. S. (1977). Perceived vulnerability and willingness to pay for crash protection. *Journal of Community Health, 3*, 136-141.

Robertston, L. S. (1981). Automobile safety regulations and death reductions in the United States. *American Journal of Public Health, 71*, 818-822.

Robertson, L. S. (1983a). Injury epidemiology and the reduction of harm. In D. Mechanic (ed.), *Handbook of health, health care and health professions.* New York: Free Press.

Robertson, L. S. (1983b). *Injuries.* Lexington, MA: Lexington Books.

Roth, J. A. (1972). Some contingencies of the moral evaluation and control of clientele: The case of the hospital emergency service. *American Journal of Surgery, 77*, 839-856.

Simmons, N. (1984, July 14). Compliance with seat belt laws said to be low. *New York Times*.

Slouching toward air bags. (1984, July 12). *Boston Globe*.

Sudnow, D. (1978). Dead on arrival. In H. D. Schwartz & C. S Kart (eds.), *Dominant issues in medical sociology.* Reading, MA: Addison-Wesley.

Syme, S. L. & Berkman, L. F. (1981). Social class, susceptibility and sickness. In P. Conrad & R. Kern (eds.), *The Sociology of health and illness: Critical perspectives.* New York: St. Martins Press.

Teufel, W. L. & Trunkey, D. D. (1977). Trauma centers: A pragmatic approach to need, cost and staffing patterns. *Journal of the American College of Emergency Physicians, 6*, 546-551.

Transport Canada. (1982). *1982: Canadian motor vehicle traffic accident statistics.* Ottawa: Transport Canada.

Trunkey, D. D. (1983a). Trauma. *Scientific American, 249*, 28-35.

Trunkey, D. D. (1983b). Predicting the community's needs: Local solutions to local problems. In J. G. West, A. B. Gazzaniga & R. H. Cales (eds.), *Trauma care systems.* New York: Praeger.

U.S. Bureau of the Census. (1982). *Statistical abstract of the United States: 1982-83* (103rd ed.). Washington, DC: Dept. of Commerce.

U.S. Bureau of the Census. (1983). *Statistical abstract of the United States: 1983-84* (104th ed.). Washington, DC: Dept. of Commerce.

U.S. Department of Health, Education and Welfare. (1979). *Healthy people.* Washington, DC: U.S. Government Printing Office.

U.S. Department of Transportation. (1984, July 17). *Fact sheet: Child passenger safety.* Washington, DC: Office of the Secretary of Transportation.

U.S. Department of Transportation. (1984, July 11). *Fact sheet: Federal motor vehicle safety standard 208, occupant crash protection.* Washington, DC: Office of the Secretary of Transportation.

U.S. Department of Transportation. (1984, July 11). *News release: Dole calls for occupant protection in cars beginning in 1986; Urges state seat belt laws.* Washington, DC: Office of Public Affairs.

Waitzkin, H. (1983). A Marxist view of health and health care. In D. Mechanic (ed.), *Handbook of health, health care and health professions*. New York: Free Press.

Waitzkin, H. (1983). *The second sickness*. New York: Free Press.

Warner, K. E. (1982). *Technology and handicapped people: Background paper #1: Mandatory passive restraint systems in automobiles: Issues and evidence*. Washington, DC: Office of Technology Assessment.

Warner, K. E. (1983). Bags, buckles and belts: The debate over mandatory passive restraints in automobiles. *Journal of Health, Policy and Law, 8*, 44-75.

Watson, G. S., Zador, P. L. & Wilks, A. (1981). Helmet use, helmet use laws, and motorcyclist fatalities. *American Journal of Public Health, 71*, 297-300.

West, J. G., Trunkey, D. D. & Lim, R. C. (1979). Systems of trauma care. *Archives of Surgery, 114*, 455-460.

West, J. G., Gazzaniga, A. B. & Cales, R. H. (eds.) (1983). *Trauma care systems: Clinical, financial considerations*. New York: Praeger.

Wikler, D. I. (1978). Persuasion and coercion for health: Ethical issues in government efforts to change lifestyles. *Milbank Memorial Fund Quarterly/Health and Society, 56*, 303-338.

Will, G. (1977, April 14). Driving without restraint. *Washington Post*.

Williams, A. F. (1979). Evaluation of the Tennessee child restraint law. *American Journal of Public Health, 69*, 455-458.

Williams, A. F., Karpf, R. S. & Zador, P. L. (1983). Variations in minimum licensing age and fatal motor vehicle crashes. *American Journal of Public Health, 73*, 1401-1403.

Williams, A. F. & Wells, J. K. (1981). The Tennessee child restraint law in its third year. *American Journal of Public Health, 71*, 163-165.

Williams, M. (1983). The trauma center designation process. In J. G. West, A. B. Gazzanga & R. H. Cales (eds.), *Trauma care systems*. New York: Praeger.

Yankauer, A. (1981). Deregulation and the right to live. *American Journal of Public Health, 71*, 797-798.

The Effectiveness of
a Self-Teaching Asthma
Self-Management Training Program
for School Age Children
and Their Families

Jonathan H. Weiss
Senior Consultant
American Lung Association

Jared A. Hermalin
Hahnemann University
and
Consultant
American Lung Association

SUMMARY. This study tested the hypothesis that an inexpensive, self-teaching asthma management training program, usable in the home environment, will be well received and prove beneficial to children with asthma and their families. A total of 321 subject families were recruited at 13 sites across the country to participate in the one year longitudinal study of the SUPERSTUFF program. Children ranged in age from 5-12, and their families constituted a heterogenous cross-section of the population. The impact of the SUPERSTUFF program was studied in relation to five major dependent variables: asthma knowledge, self-concept, asthma-related problems, asthma attitudes, and school attendance patterns. The results supported the hypothesis.

Asthma is the leading cause of chronic illness in children below the age of 17 according to the U.S. National Health Survey. Asthma heads the list of chronic illness causes of school absenteeism (NIAID, 1979), produces significant activity restrictions and adjust-

The authors wish to thank the American Lung Association, the thirteen local Lung Associations, and the 321 subject families who participated in this project. We also thank Elizabeth Konowal for her assistance in coding and computer programming. Reprints may be obtained from Jonathan H. Weiss, American Lung Association, 1740 Broadway, New York, NY 10019.

ment problems (Freudenberg, Feldman, Clark, Millman, Valle & Wasilewski, 1980; Pless & Pinkerton, 1975) and is associated with high, often excessive, use of emergency medical care (Green, Werlin, Schauffler & Avery, 1977), especially by low income families.

Asthma cannot be cured at this time. Its course, however, can be significantly influenced by medical and behavioral interventions. Among the latter, prevention programs that wed self-management practices and aggressive medical intervention have been shown to lead to: (a) better management of the illness at home; (b) fewer secondary complications (e.g., activity restrictions); (c) reduced reliance on emergency medical care; and (d) in some instances, reduced symptom frequency or severity and lowered medication costs (Green, Goldstein & Parker, 1983). Such programs typically require participants to be trained over a period of time in either a hospital, a doctor's office, a classroom, or an asthma camp. The teaching is done by professional trainers. While these characteristics contribute to the effectiveness of the programs, they are, paradoxically, the source of significant limitations. For one thing, the facilities and expertise required to mount them are not widely available, particularly in rural areas where they are especially needed. For another, they are not always well attended. In a program designed for the inner city poor, for example, fewer than 50% of enrolled families attended as many as half the sessions (Feldman & Clark, 1981), despite the fact that the same families expressed enthusiasm about exchanging knowledge, support and home management techniques in the group (Freudenberg, 1981–1982). The reasons for the low attendance figures probably include inconvenience, cost and duration of commitment, variables that have been observed repeatedly to undermine compliance to treatment regimens (Janis, 1983).

In an effort to promote prevention strategies among the millions of families with asthmatic children who are beyond the reach of professionally administered programs, or who are unable or unwilling to take advantage of such programs, the American Lung Association targeted asthma as a major focus of its education efforts in the 1980s. The Association decided to develop a self-management training program that could, if necessary, be used by patients and their families at home with minimal or no outside support. The program was to be inexpensive to purchase, easy to distribute (even in rural communities), self-motivating and self-teaching. The target audience was the elementary school age child with asthma and his/her parents. The program came to be called SUPERSTUFF.

The context for development of SUPERSTUFF had already been well established. Developing, evaluating, and disseminating self-management education programs had absorbed the efforts of a significant number of workers in the area of childhood asthma since about the mid-1970s (Green, Goldstein & Parker, 1983). Federal support for this work had been spurred, in part, by the recognition that important advances in the treatment of asthma were not being sufficiently widely used (Krause, 1983; Lenfant, 1983) and the conviction of political leaders (e.g., Bumpers, 1984) that preventive health care was not only a basic right of all Americans, but an immediate necessity for the 4,000,000 or more children (including non-asthmatics) of poor families who have no identifiable source of medical care.

In addition to government funding, foundation and nonprofit agency support for self-management training programs had also been growing. The American Lung Association was well positioned to participate in this effort by virtue of its expertise in developing and marketing educational materials for people with respiratory diseases, its visibility and credibility as a source of asthma information, and its network of affiliated Lung Associations that interface with communities and professional agencies across the country.

The SUPERSTUFF program that was developed by the senior author in collaboration with the staff of the American Lung Association and consultants from the American Thoracic Society includes: facts and myths about asthma; how to discover and avoid asthma precipitants; how to spot the early warning signs of asthma and how to deal with them effectively; relaxation, abdominal breathing warm-up exercises; and how to work more effectively with the doctor.

Throughout SUPERSTUFF there is an emphasis on competence and self-efficacy. Thus, parents and families are continuously reminded in a variety of ways that they *can* play an active role in avoiding and/or controlling asthma attacks; that they *can* be active participants in the medical management of asthma; and that they *can* contribute significantly to both the physical and psychological well-being of the asthmatic child.

Preliminary studies of SUPERSTUFF, undertaken either as a part of the development process (Whitman & Bashook, 1981) or by local Lung Associations (Knudson, 1983; Rakos, Grodek & Mack,

1983), suggested that SUPERSTUFF can be easily distributed, that it is accepted with enthusiasm, and that it is used with preventive benefits to patients and families.

The study to be reported here is the first longitudinal assessment of the effectiveness of SUPERSTUFF to be conducted on a national sample. The project was begun in September 1982 and concluded in October 1983. We evaluated the utility of SUPERSTUFF in: (a) decreasing asthma-related problems, (b) enhancing positive attitudes toward asthma, (c) increasing the patient's self-concept and knowledge of the disorder, as well as (d) decreasing the number of school days missed during the academic year. In addition, evaluation was conducted to determine the level of difficulty, interest, and continued use of SUPERSTUFF.

METHOD

Participants

Thirteen Lung Associations volunteered to participate in the one year evaluation of SUPERSTUFF. Each Association drew upon its contacts (hospitals, school nurses, HMOs, clinics, and physicians) to obtain referrals for the study. Potential subject families were contacted by the Associations and informed about the nature and duration of the study. They were assured that confidentiality would be maintained and that the study team would in no way influence their child's medical care.

Families wishing to participate in the study had to have an elementary school age asthmatic child who did not have any prior experience with SUPERSTUFF or any other formal asthma self-management training program. Families had to sign a release to obtain medical information from their physician so that the study team could confirm the asthma diagnosis. They also signed a letter of consent permitting schools to release records that would enable the study team to examine attendance patterns during the year of the study and the two previous years.

Cumulatively, 321 families participated in the study. Table 1 shows the distribution of subjects by participating Lung Associations. Northern Ohio, Kansas, Philadelphia/Montgomery County, Rhode Island, and Chicago were the top five ranked Associations in terms of their contributions to the study sample.

Table 1

Sample Distribution By ALA Service Area and

Treatment Group

Association	Experimental (n=170)	Control (n=151)	Total (n=321)
Central Indiana	5	4	9
Chicago	12	14	26
Finger Lakes	8	7	15
Iowa	7	6	13
Kansas	20	22	42
Lehigh Valley	11	9	20
Northern Ohio	29	23	52
Northwestern Ohio	6	12	18
Oregon	11	14	25
Philadelphia/Montgomery Co.	24	16	40
Rhode Island	17	15	32
San Francisco	15	3	18
Southeastern Massachusetts	5	6	11

Procedure

Participating families were assigned by random event to either an Experimental group ($n = 170$) or Control group ($n = 151$). Table 1 shows the number of subjects in each of these groups by Lung Association. Examination indicated that the groups were well matched on sociodemographic (e.g., race, age, sex of the child, years of father's education, total family income) and clinical (e.g., physician's rating of asthma severity, number of emergency room visits and number of days in hospital during the previous year) variables.

Families in the Experimental group received SUPERSTUFF by mail immediately after group assignment. The Control group did not receive SUPERSTUFF until six months into the twelve-month study. Ideally, Control group families would not have gotten SUPERSTUFF at all. It was anticipated, however, that these families would show a high drop-out rate if they were not provided an incentive for remaining.

The design of the study permitted the following longitudinal comparisons on the key dependent variables:

1. Experimental group vs. Control group during first six months.
2. Experimental group at baseline with itself over the entire year.
3. Control group during the first and last six months. (In the last six months the Control group became, in effect, a second Experimental group.)
4. Control group with itself over the last six months (post-SUPERSTUFF).

All data were collected from respondents by means of mailed questionnaires. Participating Lung Associations took responsibility for mailing the appropriate survey forms to each family at the designated data collection times. Families returned the forms to the local Lung Associations where they were checked for completeness and appropriate responses. Once verified, they were forwarded to the central data management office for computer analysis.

Measures

Basic Information Questionnaire (BIQ)

At the inception of the study, all participating families were asked to complete a 47-item scale covering demographic and disease characteristics, management issues, and known symptom precipitants. The information obtained from the BIQ enabled the research team to draw a profile of the total sample as well as to examine the match of the Experimental and Control groups when these were constituted.

Test-retest reliability for items involving recall (e.g., number of days lost from work because of the child's asthma) showed 64% perfect agreement, 17% partial agreement (defined as less than a 20% discrepancy) and 19% disagreement.

Asthma Problem Checklist (APCL)

The Asthma Problem Checklist (APCL) consists of a series of eight subscales, each concerned with a different asthma-related problem. These include problems related to the use of medicine (11 items); early signs of asthma (5); triggers of asthma (10); child's behavior during an attack (9); behavior of other's during an attack (8); asthma effects on social development (8); asthma effects on school (5); and asthma effects on the family (6). Subtotals for each subscale were computed as well as an overall, cumulative total. Item scores ranged from 0 (never a problem) to 4 (always a problem). The checklist was completed by the parent.

The APCL was developed at the National Asthma Center. It has a reported test-retest reliability in excess of .90. Our own reliability check showed comparable results. Internal consistency of the APCL is reflected in correlation coefficients ranging from .66 to .77 between the eight subscale scores and the total problems score, and subscale intercorrelations ranging from .3 to .5 (Creer, Marion & Creer, 1983).

Asthma Attitude Scales (AAS)

Parent's Scale. The Parent's Scale consists of a series of 24 questions, divided into two subscales (C & D), the former containing 18 items, the latter six. The C scale focuses primarily on attitudes covering what the child and adult can do to manage the asthma disorder. The D scale focuses on the asthmatic's relationship to the outside world. For each, the most positive response is scored a 4, the most negative a 0.

Child's Scale. The Child's Scale consists of a series of 28 questions, divided into two subscales (C & S_c), the former containing 12 items, the latter 16. The C scale is concerned with what the child can do about the asthma condition. The S_c scale relates to how asthma impacts on one's perceptions of self and interaction with others. Scoring is as in the Parent's Scale.

Both Asthma Attitude Scales, as well as the Asthma Problem Checklist, were developed by Thomas L. Creer of the National Asthma Center.

Piers-Harris Self-Concept Inventory (SCI)

This inventory consists of 80 questions related to the "way I feel about myself." Each positive response scored one point, each negative response 0 points. The form was completed by the child, with parental assistance. Norms were based on 1183 public school children ranging from grades 4-12 (Piers & Harris, 1969).

Asthma Knowledge Test (AKT)

The test comprises a total of 24 questions covering crucial areas of asthma addressed in SUPERSTUFF. Each correct response scored one point, each incorrect response 0 points. Eight questions allowed for more than one correct response. This form was completed by the parent. Test-retest reliability showed that there was 67% perfect agreement, 13% partial agreement (on items where more than one answer was possible) and 20% disagreement between answers.

SUPERSTUFF Evaluation Questionnaire

The questionnaire consisted of two forms, both completed by parents.

Form A. This form consisted of nine questions related to how SUPERSTUFF affected asthma management; whether the child was taking greater responsibility for the asthma condition; whether the family was more confident and less worried about the disorder; and whether parental relationships with the child had improved since receiving SUPERSTUFF.

Form B. This form consisted of 13 questions related to interest in SUPERSTUFF, difficulty of the materials, and degree and longevity of their use.

Table 2 demonstrates the data collection points for each of the measures.

Since a substantial amount of baseline information was requested, data collection was spread out over a two month period: September-October 1982. Included were the Background Information Questionnaire, Asthma Problem Checklist, Asthma Attitude Scales, the Piers-Harris Self-Concept Inventory, and Asthma Knowledge Test.

To allow for multiple Experimental-Control group comparisons during the first six months, the Problem Checklist, Self-Concept Inventory, and Asthma Knowledge Test were obtained from both groups at four and six months.

Following the six-month data collection period, the Control group received SUPERSTUFF. Analysis then shifted toward Control group assessment pre- and post-SUPERSTUFF, as well as longer-term testing of SUPERSTUFF on the Experimental group. For the Controls, eight- and eleven-month scores on the Problem Checklist and Self-Concept Inventory were compared to the latest pre-SUPERSTUFF scores taken at six months. Asthma Knowledge Test scores at eight months were also compared to the six-month scores. For the Experimental group, the twelve-month follow-up on

Table 2

Data Collection Schedule

	Baseline[a]	4 Months Exp	4 Months Con	6 Months[b] Exp	6 Months[b] Con	8 Months Exp	8 Months Con	11 Months Exp	11 Months Con	12 Months Exp	12 Months Con
Basic Information Questionnaire	X										
Problem Checklist	X	X	X	X	X		X		X	X	
Asthma Attitude Scales											
Adult	X	X	X	X	X	X			X		
Child	X	X	X	X	X	X			X		
Self-Concept Inventory	X	X	X	X	X		X		X		
Asthma Knowledge Test	X	X	X	X	X		X				
Evaluation											
Form A		X	X	X	X		X		X	X	
Form B		X	X	X	X		X		X	X	
Attendance Data[c]										X	X

[a] Experimental group received SUPERSTUFF after submitting baseline survey.

[b] Control group received SUPERSTUFF after submitting 6-month follow-up survey.

[c] Attendance data for the first two years were submitted by the school at their convenience; all three years had to be submitted by the last follow-up.

the eight Problem Checklist measures was similarly related to six-month scores.

Asthma Attitude Scales were not collected as often as the above variables because it was felt that a longer experience with the materials would be necessary before attitude changes were likely to occur. Thus, for the Experimental group, AAS follow-up at eight months was compared to the baseline report; for the Controls, five-month post-SUPERSTUFF scores (obtained during the eleventh month of the study) were compared to baseline reports.

Evaluation data were collected from Experimental subjects at four, six, and twelve months; from the Controls at two and five months post-SUPERSTUFF (the eighth and eleventh study months).

School attendance data were obtained for the year of the study and for the two previous years, for both Experimental and Control subjects. It was hypothesized that there would be no difference between the two groups in the two years before the study (as SUPERSTUFF had not yet been introduced) but that in the third year the Experimental group would do significantly better. (The Controls did not receive SUPERSTUFF until near the end of the school year.)

Program

The wide array of dependent variables described above were selected for study because of the broad scope of the SUPERSTUFF program. Like the professionally administered programs, SUPER-STUFF emphasizes cognition (e.g., scientific understanding of asthma rather than folklore), performance (e.g., avoidance of precipitants, effectively dealing with early warning signs of an attack), affect (e.g., relaxation) and cooperation (e.g., between family members, as well as between family and medical personnel). SUPERSTUFF seeks to: dispel myths about asthma; provide answers to commonly asked questions about the disorder; educate children and parents about typical precipitants and warning signs; help individual families to discover the specific noxious agents that precipitate their child's attacks; teach children how to breathe and relax so as to ward off or minimize an oncoming attack; teach effective ways to communicate with medical staff; and build the self-esteem and confidence of the asthmatic child.

SUPERSTUFF, as mentioned above, is a program whose use is independent of support from outside sources. To make the program self-motivating, its format was chosen to be both familiar and attractive to the target group at which it was aimed, viz., children 6-12 years old and their parents. It was also designed in a fashion that would maximize the probability of continued use. The children's manual is an 86 page "book" in full color, containing games, stickers, models, stories, puzzles, etc., that children in that age range do with pleasure. The parents' module is an informal news magazine called, "How To Control Asthma." It is written in non-technical language and richly illustrated. In designing the materials we were careful not to imply, in any sense, that having asthma is fun. We saw no reason, however, why learning about its management should not be fun, especially if that would help to reach and hold the interest of the young child. In both the children's and parents' modules serious information is presented, whenever possible, in a lighthearted, upbeat manner.

An important objective of SUPERSTUFF was to defuse asthma, making children and adults less embarrassed and ashamed of it. Thus, stickers and a large colorful SUPERSTUFF poster were included to encourage the child to "go public"; not to feel alone and different. It was hoped that in the process of doing so the child would also come to feel better about him/herself.

The information and techniques described in SUPERSTUFF suggest certain competencies users should not only acquire, but be aware that they possess. Phrases such as "I control," "I know," or "I understand" recur in the materials several times, in order to encourage a sense of self-efficacy and control (Weiss, 1981). Too many children and adults are overwhelmed by asthma because they have not been helped to realize that they *can* participate in the prevention and control of symptom episodes.

RESULTS

Before describing the results of the study a word is in order about attrition. The overall retention rate by the end of the study was approximately 65%. This figure is, however, not very informative because it was not representative. Lung Associations varied as widely in retention rates as they did in recruitment figures, with the most successful Associations retaining as much as 85% of their samples for the duration of the study. This variability was, so far as we were able to tell, a function of the variable amount of resources that Associations could commit to support the project. Associations with small staffs raised fewer participant families and, in many instances, were able to follow fewer of them closely enough to keep them in the study.

SUPERSTUFF Evaluation Questionnaire

Form A

For the Experimental group, a sizeable percentage of parents reported positive gains as early as three months post-SUPER-STUFF. As an illustration, at three months 66% of responding parents reported an improvement in their management of the child's asthma. By 12 months, this figure was 79%. Similarly, 69% of respondents judged their child's management of the asthma to have been improved within the first three months; 87% gave this reply at 12 months. In terms of confidence, 77% of respondents in the Experimental group indicated greater confidence in asthma management at three months, and 87% gave this report at the last reporting period. Seventy-five and 84% of responding parents reported their children's confidence had increased during the corresponding time periods. Somewhat of a surprise was the immediate effect SUPERSTUFF was reported to have had on the parent-child relationship: 51% of respondents reported an improved relationship by the third month after receiving SUPERSTUFF. (This figure remained relatively constant throughout the year.) Control group reports, following receipt of SUPERSTUFF, were comparable to those of the Experimental group.

Form B

At the first follow-up, 60% of the Experimental group parents indicated their children's reaction to SUPERSTUFF was enthusiastic. By the end of 12 months, 54% of respondents judged their children to be still feeling this way. A total of 84% of Experimental group respondents believed the materials were about right for their child's reading abilities; 97% believed this about the parent's magazine. By the 12th month, 66% still found the parent's magazine very interesting. Of particular importance was the fact that more than 80% of the children who were reported to have had asthma attacks since getting the materials were said to have used

SUPERSTUFF suggestions to control those episodes, indicating that the SUPERSTUFF approach had become an integral part of their asthma management strategy. (Control group results, post-SUPERSTUFF, were again comparable.)

School Attendance

No significant differences were found between the Experimental and Control groups during the two school years prior to the study when examination was made of (a) the absolute number of school days in attendance; and (b) the proportionate days in attendance. During the study year, however, the analysis of variance test demonstrated that Experimental group children attended significantly more days than the Controls (167.55 vs. 162.80, $F = 5.78$, $p < .02$), a difference of a full school week. In terms of proportionate days in attendance, the result was also significant (.942 vs. .913, $F = 8.38$, $p < .005$). These results supported the dual hypotheses: (a) there would be no significant differences between the randomly designed groups pre-SUPERSTUFF; and (b) the Experimental group would do better during the study year, following exposure to the SUPERSTUFF program.

Asthma Attitude Scales

For each of the attitudes scales, separate t-tests were calculated for the Experimental and Control groups because of the disparity in data collection periods.

In the Experimental group, the child's mean $(\bar{X})$ total attitude score $(C + S_c)$ showed significant gains from baseline (t_1) to follow-up at 8 months (t_8), $(\bar{X}_1 = 82.00, \bar{X}_8 = 87.86, t = 3.80, p < .001)$. The child's C sub-scale score (which relates to the child's taking positive steps toward dealing with the asthmatic condition) also showed significant gains $(\bar{X}_1 = 31.39, \bar{X}_8 = 38.42, t = 8.91, p < .001)$. There were no significant changes in adult attitudes.

For the Control group (compared pre- vs. post-SUPERSTUFF), the child's mean total attitude score demonstrated significant gains. At baseline (t_1), the mean was 87.57. In the 11th month (i.e., five months after receipt of SUPERSTUFF) the mean was 91.21 $(t = 2.28, p < .03)$. The S_c scale (which relates to perceptions of self and others) also showed advances in a positive direction $(\bar{X}_1 = 53.04, \bar{X}_{11} = 55.30, t = 2.51, p < .02)$, while the C subscale demonstrated a trend ($\bar{X}_1 = 34.23$, $\bar{X}_{11} = 35.84$, $t = 1.81$, $p < .08$) in the appropriate direction.

Unlike what was seen in the Experimental group, adult Control group scores showed significant changes: (a) the total score ($\bar{X}_1 = 79.59$, $\bar{X}_{11} = 82.06$, $t = 3.22$, $p < .002$); (b) the C subscale score, what the child and adult can do to manage the asthma ($\bar{X}_1 = 58.57$, $\bar{X}_{11} = 59.90$, $t = 2.08$, $p < .05$); and (c) the D scale score, the asthmatic's relationship to the outside world ($\bar{X}_1 = 21.24$, $\bar{X}_{11} = 22.26$, $t = 4.06$, $p < .001$) all changed in a positive direction.

SCI, AKT, and APCL

For the remaining three outcome measures, SCI, AKT, and APCL, comparisons were made between the Experimental and Control groups during the first six months of the study, using baseline scores as covariates (to partial out any baseline differences). In all analyses of variance the effects of asthma severity and father's education were examined. Severity was selected as a factor for examination because it might be expected to influence perception of the problem, management issues, need for further knowledge about the disorder, and feelings of self. Father's education was selected because it is a variable that, in other studies, has been shown to be a major determinant of receptivity to and use of educational programs. In the present study it would be expected that families with lower father's education level would report less use of the SUPERSTUFF principles and greater asthma problem prevalence, have lower knowledge test scores, and score poorer on the self-concept scale.

Father's education was dichotomized at less than or equal to completion of high school (≤ 12 years) and completion of at least one year of college (> 13 years). Asthma severity, based on the physician's rating, was dichotomized at low to mild and moderate to severe/refractory.

Self-Concept

Comparisons between Experimental and Control groups could be made during the first six months of the study, because data were collected for both groups at baseline, four, and six months. Experimental and Control group subjects all showed positive increases despite the fact that the Control group had not yet received SUPERSTUFF. At both four and six months, there were no significant differences between the two groups, after covarying their baseline differences.

To assess pre-post SUPERSTUFF changes in the Control group, comparisons were made between (a) six- and eight-month scores and (b) six- and eleven-month scores. In both instances, there were significant increases in self-concept ($\bar{X}_6 = 65.19$, $\bar{X}_8 = 67.46$, $F = 5.37$, $p < .03$; $\bar{X}_6 = 65.33$, $\bar{X}_{11} = 70.04$, $F = 15.87$, $p < .01$).

Asthma Knowledge Test

Controlling for baseline scores, the Experimental group showed significantly higher mean AKT scores than the Controls at four months post-SUPERSTUFF (27.34 vs. 26.53, $F = 4.12$, $p < .05$). This suggested that even at the first follow-up the program may have had an impact on asthma knowledge. When, however, father's education and severity were examined as additional factors, the significant difference was found to be attributable to father's education, not SUPERSTUFF (High Educ. = 27.79, Low Educ. = 26.69, $F = 6.53$, $p < .02$). High education fathers had higher knowledge test scores.

At six months post-SUPERSTUFF the same pattern held. SUPERSTUFF was still not demonstrating significance while father's education continued to do so (High Educ. = 27.94, Low Educ. = 26.10, $F = 7.11$, $p < .01$) and in the same direction.

When comparing the control group to itself at six and eight months (pre- and post-SUPERSTUFF), a significant interaction between knowledge and father's education was revealed ($F = 5.81$, $p < .02$). Knowledge mean scores increased during this period, with father's education contributing to this effect.

Asthma Problem Checklist

The APCL is composed of eight subscales, each addressed at multiple periods of time. Experimental subjects were asked to respond to the eight measures at baseline, four, six, and twelve months. Controls were asked to respond at baseline, four, six, eight, and eleven months.

Because the Controls received SUPERSTUFF only after the six-month follow-up, we compared them with the Experimental subjects until that time. We hypothesized that the Experimentals would do significantly better on all problem measures.

After the sixth month, the effects of SUPERSTUFF on the

Control group were analyzed by comparing post-SUPERSTUFF scores (eight and eleven months) with pre-SUPERSTUFF scores (six months). In similar fashion, Experimental group scores at twelve months were compared with six-month scores to determine whether there was a continuing SUPERSTUFF impact beyond the first half year.

Four-Month Follow-Up

At this first follow-up comparison point, three significant or trend ($p < .10$) differences emerged when SUPERSTUFF treatment (Experimental vs. Control placement), father's education, and asthma severity were examined as factors. Only one of these was in the predicted direction, demonstrating a minimal short-term impact of the SUPERSTUFF program on APCL.

Other's Behavior During an Attack. A significant interaction effect was found with SUPERSTUFF treatment, father's education, and asthma severity ($F = 4.50, p < .04$). The Experimental group of low education and high severity demonstrated lower mean problem scores than comparable Controls (2.08 vs. 3.41).

School Problems. A significant interaction effect was found with treatment, education and severity ($F = 5.87, p < .02$). The Experimental group of higher education and high severity demonstrated greater mean problem scores than comparable Controls (3.79 vs. 2.54).

Medication Use. A trend interaction effect was found between treatment, education and severity ($F = 3.84, p < .06$). Experimental group subjects of low severity and high education were shown to have higher mean medical problem scores than comparable Controls (6.82 vs. 4.84).

Six-Month Follow-Up

At the second follow-up, five significant/trend results were observed.

School Problems. A significant main effect was found as a function of treatment ($F = 6.41, p < .02$). Experimental group subjects demonstrated lower mean school problem scores when compared to Controls (2.96 vs. 4.01).

Early Signs. A significant interaction effect was found with treatment and severity ($F = 8.50, p < .01$). The Experimental group of high severity showed lower mean sign problems than comparable Controls (4.35 vs. 6.44).

Triggers. A significant interaction effect was found with treatment and severity ($F = 6.14$, $p < .02$). The high severity Experimental group exhibited lower mean trigger problems than comparable Controls (14.42 vs. 16.41).

Family Problems. A trend interaction effect was found with treatment and severity ($F = 3.43$, $p < .07$). Experimental subjects of high severity demonstrated lower mean family problem scores than comparable Controls (2.27 vs. 3.14).

Medication Use. A trend interaction effect was found with treatment and severity ($F = 3.08$, $p < .09$). High severity Experimental subjects reported lower mean medication problem scores than comparable Controls (6.19 vs. 8.17).

By the sixth month, then, SUPERSTUFF effects on APCL were becoming apparent.

Eight-Month Follow-Up

The reader will recall that after the six-month data collection period, the Control group received SUPERSTUFF. From this time on, therefore, analyses were conducted separately for Experimental and Control groups. Results reported here are from comparisons of Controls pre- versus post-SUPERSTUFF (i.e., at six and eight months).

School Problems. A significant main effect was found ($F = 6.30$, $p < .02$). The Control group reported lower mean school problem scores in the eighth as compared to the sixth month (3.25 vs. 3.92). This supports the hypothesis of lower problem scores following exposure to SUPERSTUFF.

Early Signs. A significant interaction effect was found between signs and severity ($F = 6.28$, $p < .02$). The prevalence of sign problems decreased between the sixth and eighth month, again supporting the hypothesis. Higher severity was also related to more problems, as might be expected.

Total Problems. A significant main effect was found with father's education ($F = 7.35$, $p < .01$). The higher father's education level, the greater the mean total problem score reported (High Educ. = 52.53, Low Educ. = 33.64). This was contrary to our expectation.

Triggers. A significant main effect was found with father's education ($F = 4.78$, $p < .04$). Again, the higher father's education level, the greater the mean trigger problems reported (High Educ. = 16.32, Low Educ. = 12.75).

Child's Behavior During an Attack. A significant main effect was found with father's education ($F = 8.09, p < .01$). Once more, the higher father's education level the greater the prevalence of problems reported (High Educ. = 7.56, Low Educ. = 4.14).

Eleven-Month Follow-Up: Control Group

For the Controls, comparisons were made between the sixth and eleventh months. The reader should keep in mind that at this follow-up the Controls had been exposed to SUPERSTUFF for five months, approximately the amount of time at which the positive impact of SUPERSTUFF was most prominent in the Experimental group.

Development Problems. A significant main effect was found ($F = 6.47, p < .02$). The Control group reported fewer developmental problems in the eleventh as compared to the sixth month (3.71 vs. 4.64). This finding supports the SUPERSTUFF hypothesis.

Family Problems. A trend main effect was found ($F = 3.63, p < .07$). There was a tendency toward fewer problems in the eleventh month (2.14 vs. 2.51) further suggesting a positive effect of SUPERSTUFF.

Problem Total. A trend main effect was found ($F = 3.59, p < .07$). There was a trend toward fewer problems overall in the eleventh, as compared to the sixth, month (44.51 vs. 48.36). Again this is in the predicted direction.

Early Warning Signs. A significant main effects were found with father's education ($F = 6.40, p < .02$) and severity ($F = 6.15, p < .02$). Both high education and high severity are related to higher mean early warning sign problems (5.62 vs. 3.52; 5.65 vs. 3.80, respectively). The latter is in the expected direction. The former, however, is contrary to expectation.

Twelve-Month Follow-Up: Experimental Group

Comparisons between the sixth and twelfth months revealed three significant/trend effects. None clearly supported the SUPERSTUFF hypothesis, however.

Early Warning Signs. A significant main effect was found ($F = 6.26, p < .02$). There was an apparent regression toward the mean as the prevalence of sign problems was greater in the twelfth than in the sixth month (5.41 vs. 4.59).

Triggers. A significant interaction effect was found between triggers and severity ($F = 6.37$, $p < .02$). Low severity children showed a decrease in problems between the sixth and twelfth months, while high severity children demonstrated an increase during the same time period.

Medication Use. A trend interaction effect was found between medication use, father's education and severity ($F = 3.40$, $p < .08$). High education, low severity children indicated a greater prevalence of problems in the twelfth month than in the sixth month (6.86 vs. 5.86). Low education, low severity children manifested a lower prevalence of medication problems in the twelfth month (6.08 vs. 7.92).

DISCUSSION

The results reported above, taken in concert, suggest that the premise upon which the development of SUPERSTUFF was based, i.e., that a self-teaching asthma self-management training program would be well received and used with subsequent benefits, is essentially correct. Parents in the study reported that SUPERSTUFF was used by them and their children with enthusiasm and that a variety of benefits followed. Experimental group children attended significantly more school days during the year of the follow-up than did Control children. Changes that were detected on the Asthma Attitude and Self-Concept scales were in the desired direction. Changes on the Asthma Problem Checklist were also, on the whole, in the direction of fewer problems post-SUPERSTUFF.

Nevertheless, with few exceptions, the magnitude of changes was not large. In evaluating the meaning of this fact, it should be recalled that no attempt was made to select subjects for the study who might have been expected to differentially benefit from asthma self-management training. All volunteers with a confirmed diagnosis of asthma were included. The resulting sample was knowledgeable about asthma and relatively problem free even before SUPERSTUFF. On the whole, SUPERSTUFF was tested on a sample for whom ceiling effects appear to have restricted the amount of change that could be observed. Nonetheless, we did observe a number of significant changes. In other studies of hospital-based training programs it has been observed that post-training effects (e.g., reduced emergency room visits) are more pronounced in children who have had more room to change (i.e., had more emergency room visits during the previous year). Had we limited our sample to more severely ill children with more pronounced asthma problems, emergency room usage, etc., more substantial changes might have been observed.

A finding on the SUPERSTUFF Evaluation Questionnaire that is worth special note relates to the reported longevity of use of the materials. In the original validation study of SUPERSTUFF conducted at Michael Reese Medical Center, it was concluded that the materials would arouse great initial interest that would dissipate within several weeks. The results of the present study, however, show that after as much as a year, 40% of the asthmatic children in respondent families still continue to express an interest in SUPER-STUFF despite their young age, and 80% of those children who had experienced symptom episodes are still utilizing SUPERSTUFF suggestions or information in time of need. For those families it would appear that SUPERSTUFF and self-management had become a part of the armamentarium of techniques for coping with asthma. This finding encourages us to believe that the efforts required to promote and distribute SUPERSTUFF result in gains that are not merely transitory. We, therefore, recommend that SUPERSTUFF be distributed to all pediatric asthma patients for home use.

The reader may have noted that father's education level was a significant factor in the Asthma Knowledge Test and Asthma Problem Checklist analyses. With regard to the AKT, higher education was associated with higher knowledge test scores, an expectable result. With regard to the APCL, the results were more complex. Among the findings, one consistent pattern appeared in the scores of the Control group post-SUPERSTUFF. Higher education was associated with *higher* problem scores, contrary to what was expected. The interpretation offered is that more educated families were more receptive to SUPERSTUFF, as we expected, and that with the knowledge they acquired, they became more aware of problems that went unnoticed by the low education families (who may either have used the materials less diligently or applied the information contained therein less often). It is also possible that having used SUPER-STUFF, higher education level families set higher standards of control and were, therefore, more wary and inclined to report problems than were their lower education counterparts.

It is necessary to consider the problem of sample attrition on the meaning of our findings. As mentioned above, approximately 65% of our sample was retained through the year of the study. Is it possible, then, that the positive changes over time are merely apparent and reflect only the changing composition of our groups as more "negative" families dropped out? We believe that there are three arguments against this possibility. First, attrition varied greatly across participating Lung Associations and was tied primarily to the resources that each Association was able to allocate to the study. (There was no funding to participating sites. All efforts were donated voluntarily.) If attrition was an index of (negative) attitude toward SUPERSTUFF and, thus, a confounding variable, one would expect to find the most positive findings in Associations which experienced the highest attrition rates. An examination of our data revealed no such systematic pattern. Second, our school absenteeism data are our most objective measurements and were provided by schools, not by parents. In fact, in a number of instances school absenteeism data were obtained for children whose families had already dropped from the study. And third, the regression of the Experimental group's APCL scores toward the end of the year argues against a simple attrition-induced bias toward more positive scores over time.

Finally, a comment is in order about the generalizability of our findings. An examination of the sociodemographic and clinical background of our sample reveals that there was diversity in age, sex, ethnicity, religion, income, parents' education, history of asthma in the family, severity and measures of health care utilization. No important subgroups appear to have been excluded. We believe, therefore, that it is justified to anticipate that the gains reported by the present sample would occur in similar samples drawn at random for the asthmatic population of the United States of elementary school age. We are mindful, nevertheless, of the fact mentioned above that on a number of criteria our sample included a substantial representation of asthmatic children who scored toward the mild end of the severity continuum.

REFERENCES

Bumpers, D. (1984). Securing the blessings of liberty for posterity: Preventive health care for children. *American Psychologist, 39*, 896-900.

Creer, T. L., Marion, R. S. & Creer, P. P. (1983). Asthma Problems Behavior Checklist: Parental perceptions of the behavior of asthmatic children. *Journal of Asthma, 20*, 97-104.

Feldman, C. H. & Clark, N. M. (1981). Development and evaluation of a self-management program for children with asthma. In *Self-management education programs for childhood asthma proceedings* (Vol. 2). Center for Interdisciplinary Research in Immunological Diseases, National Institute for Allergy & Infectious Diseases, Asthma and Allergy Foundation of America.

Freudenberg, N. (1981-82). Self-help within a medical institution: Its potentials and limits. *International Quarterly of Community Health Education, 2*, 215-223.

Freudenberg, N., Feldman, C. H., Clark, N. M., Millman, E. J., Valle, I. & Wasilewski, Y. (1980). The impact of bronchial asthma on school attendance and performance. *Journal of School Health, 50*, 522-526.

Green, L. W., Goldstein, R. A. & Parker, S. R. (1983). Conclusions & recommendations. In *Self-Management of Childhood Asthma: Supplementary Issue. Journal of Allergy and Clinical Immunology, 72*.

Green, L. W., Werlin, S. H., Schauffler, H. H. & Avery, C. H. (1977). Research and demonstration issues in self-care: Measuring the decline of medico-centrism. *Health Education Monographs, 5*, 161-189.

Janis, I. (1983). The role of social support in adherence to stressful decisions. *American Psychologist, 38*, 143-160.

Karetzky, M. (1977). Asthma in the South Bronx: Clinical and epidemiological characteristics. *Journal of Allergy and Clinical Immunology, 60*, 383-390.

Knudson, S. (1983). SUPERSTUFF asthma program. Final report to the Boettcher Foundation.

Krause, R. M. (1983). Asthma self-management: Perspective from the NIAID. *Journal of Allergy and Clinical Immunology, 72*, 520-521.

Lenfant, C. J. M. (1983). Asthma self-management: Perspective from the NHLBI. *Journal of Allergy and Clinical Immunology, 72*, 521-522.

National Institute for Allergy & Infectious Diseases Task Force. (1979). *Asthma and Other Allergic Diseases*. National Institute of Health Publication #79-397.

Piers, E. V. & Harris, D. B. (1969). *The Piers-Harris Children's Self-Concept Scale*. Nashville: Counselor Recordings and Tests.

Pless, I. & Pinkerton, P. (1975). *Chronic childhood disorders promoting patterns of adjustment*. London: Henry Kempton Publishing.

Rakos, R., Grodek, M. & Mack, K. (1983). An empirical evaluation of the self-help program "SUPERSTUFF" for asthmatic children. Paper presented at the Annual Meeting of the American Thoracic Society, Kansas City, MO.

Weiss, J. H. (1981). SUPERSTUFF. In *Self-management educational programs for childhood asthma*. Proceedings of a conference sponsored by the Center for Interdisciplinary Research in Immunologic Diseases, UCLA; National Institute of Allergy and Infectious Diseases; and Asthma and Allergy Foundation of America.

Whitman, N. & Bashook, P. (1981). *Validation study of SUPERSTUFF*. Report to the American Lung Association, New York.

Prevention
and Community Compliance
to Immunization Schedules

Lizette Peterson
University of Missouri-Columbia

SUMMARY. Examples of Bloom's (1968) three methods of effecting primary prevention were utilized in a single community agency to increase community compliance to immunization regimens. A milestone approach which utilized written prompts to parents delivered by school age children and school-based clinics produced large increases in the number of children immunized, with very low cost. A community wide DHEW public service media campaign did not result in an appreciable increase in immunizations obtained, but a community wide measles epidemic and accompanying free clinics also publicized by the media resulted in large increases in the number of individuals immunized. Finally, telephone contact, but not mail contact, with parents of high risk, low socioeconomic status preschool children produced a moderate improvement in immunization status. The implications of each of these specific interventions are considered, including explicit and implicit costs and benefits for the community.

During the past decade, the public health emphasis on prevention of injury and illness has been joined by a similar emphasis in the field of health psychology. Public health interventions have typically involved population-wide contact, with environmental manipulations. Mandated safe construction of infant cribs and fluoride in drinking water are examples of such endeavors. In contrast, health psychology has attempted to intervene at the individual's level to effect lifestyle changes such as increasing compliance to dietary

Sincere appreciation is extended to Andrew L. Homer and Vanessa Selby for their comments on earlier drafts of this manuscript and to the staff of the Boone County-Columbia City Health Department for their cooperation with this research. This work was supported by a Summer Fellowship from the Research Council of the University of Missouri-Columbia. Reprints may be obtained from Lizette Peterson, Psychology Department, 210 McAlester, University of Missouri-Columbia, Columbia, MO 65211.

restrictions, pediatric health care visits, and dental procedures, and decreasing maladaptive patterns such as smoking and overeating. Peterson and Mori (1985) and Roberts, Elkins and Royal (1984) have recently reviewed both approaches and conclude that both offer important strengths for future preventive intervention. The present study focuses on some typical interventions drawn from both the public health and the health psychology areas. These interventions sought to influence an important aspect of prevention in child health—the obtaining of immunization for disease.

Compliance to suggested immunization schedules for children constitutes a major influence on community health patterns (Imperato, 1974). Indeed, some professionals have noted that a child's immunization status can serve as an indicator of the quality of the child's overall medical care (Barkin, Barkin & Roth, 1977). As such, the current trends toward lowered levels of community immunization to disease are alarming. Although the past century has heralded the possible eradication of sometimes fatal childhood diseases through the use of appropriate vaccines, the 1973 National Immunization Survey noted a significant decrease in the immunization levels among preschool children (Krugman & Katz, 1977). Not only are more children susceptible to diseases such as whooping cough, diphtheria, tetanus, measles and mumps than before, but in some cases their susceptibility will continue through adulthood and may ultimately affect their own children (Marcuse, 1975). Millions of dollars each year are lost due to diseases which could have been prevented by immunization (Mortimer, 1978). In response to such factors, former Secretary of DHEW, Joseph Califano, launched a nationwide drive during 1977-1978 to immunize at least 90% of children in the United States. However, many health experts report continued evidence of children who are underimmunized. Some health professionals have suggested that the 1977 immunization drive produced statistical gains which are not reflected in actual improvements in immunization levels within some specific target groups, particularly lower socioeconomic status children (Bergman, 1979).

A variety of methods have been used to effect compliance to immunization schedules, with differing levels of success. Increasing health education programs has typically not produced large increases in immunization (e.g., Imperato, Pincus, Hwa & Chaves, 1974) and one time prompts such as a single written reminder have not evidenced much success either (e.g., Yokley, Glenwick, Hedrick & Page, 1980). Some methods such as the use of repeated prompts in the forms of letters and phone calls have been relatively effective, but only for a "captive" population such as school-age children (e.g., Vernon, Connor, Shaw, Lampe & Doster, 1976). The use of repeated contact plus home visiting has also been demonstrated to increase immunization levels in high risk populations (Minear & Guyer, 1979), but this method has been criticized as being extremely expensive (Bergman, 1979).

In fact, many of the successful methods for increasing the rate at which individuals obtain immunization for themselves and for their children can be prohibitively expensive, both in terms of financial outlay and in terms of time demands on already overworked staff members. The extent to which prevention programs will actually be used is determined by their success and by their ease of implementation; a successful program which is unlikely to be implemented may be of very little value (Peterson & Ridley-Johnson, 1983). In the long run, decisions concerning the implementation of preventive programs may be a function of cost/benefit analyses (Rossi, Freeman & Wright, 1979), with the programs yielding the greatest benefit at the lowest cost actually being implemented. Indeed, the costs cannot be estimated entirely in terms of financial considerations; staff effort and energy may be more important aspects of implementation than financial outlay.

The formulation of programs which can not only offer some promise of success but also can be readily implemented will require innovation. Bloom (1968) outlined three major types of interventions which could be used in primary prevention, including not only (a) high risk prevention but also (b) community wide and (c) milestone preventive interventions. Milestone approaches involve preventive intervention with children as they pass through some developmental milestone or time period. Community wide approaches are typified by contact with entire communities, often through mass mailings or media.

The following two studies provide illustration of how in a single community setting, the three major types of interventions described by Bloom have been directed toward elevating community immunization levels. The first study was a quasi-experiment which utilized epidemiological data to examine milestone and community wide approaches. The present milestone approach was a statewide immunization initiative directed toward elementary school-age children, while the community wide intervention was a federal program using media based public service announcements. The second study focused on an individualized intervention with a high risk population.

STUDY 1

Method

Subjects

All those individuals living in the catchment area of the Boone County-Columbia City Health Department served as subjects (100,376 persons, 6,272 of whom were under age 5, lived in this predominantly rural catchment area of mid-Missouri during the period of this study).

Procedure

Data on the number of immunizations obtained from the Columbia Health Department were collected from January 1973 to September 1979. These data form only an estimate of the number of immunizations obtained by the community as a whole, since private practice physicians also provide immunizations. However, because the Health Department office regularly serves a very large number of individuals (estimated at 2,200 persons per year for the period of this study), and never closes for vacations or other seasonal variations, these data may provide a stable sampling for immunizations obtained within this community. This study obtained data on the occurrence of both milestone and community wide interventions. The milestone study targeted school-age children, with elementary school registration selected as an appropriate developmental event. The community wide intervention employed public service media campaigns encouraging immunizations among the entire community, both children and unimmunized adults.

At the beginning of each school year, the parents of Missouri children are reminded that by law the child must be immunized to enter school. Two milestone interventions were held during March-April 1975 and November 1977, when every elementary school in the catchment area sent reminders to the parents of enrolled children noting that by law all elementary school age children must be immunized for polio, diphtheria, tetanus, and pertussis. Parents were informed that by signing a release form their children could be immunized at a free clinic held at the school. The March-April 1975 and November 1977 interventions were the only instances of free school clinics during the course of this study. The financial cost to the Health Department of these interventions included only the cost of the vaccine, printing of the forms, and the cost of Health Department staff transportation to the schools. Community volunteers assisted at the immunization clinics, but Health Department staff provided the actual immunizations.

Two other kinds of interventions for immunization also occurred during the period of this study. These used community wide techniques. In October 1973 and August 1978 the Department of Health, Education and Welfare (DHEW, now the Department of Health and Human Services) launched nationwide advertisement campaigns designed to increase immunization levels. Public service announcements enjoining viewers to contact their physician or local health department to obtain immunizations occurred several times daily for two separate two month periods (October-November 1973, August-September 1978) on all three local television stations and were carried several times a week by local radio stations and newspapers. A second, although less programmatic, community wide intervention took place when a county wide measles epidemic occurred in May of 1977. Local news broadcasts daily noted the dangers of children and adults contracting the disease and advised immunization as a precaution, reporting on community clinics offering free immunization in a variety of locations such as schools and churches. Again, the cost of the clinics to the Health Department included the vaccine, transportation costs, and some staff overtime. The news coverage was, of course, free.

Results

Figure 1 demonstrates the total number of immunizations obtained from January 1973 to September 1979. Public concern was focused on immunization levels in the 1973 National Immunization Survey conducted by the Department of Health, Education and Welfare. Beginning at this time, there is an uneven but overall increase in immunizations given by the Health Department, as can be seen in Figure 1. The large increases in immunizations following milestone interventions are most noteworthy. As can be seen in Figure 1, following the first milestone parental prompting—the

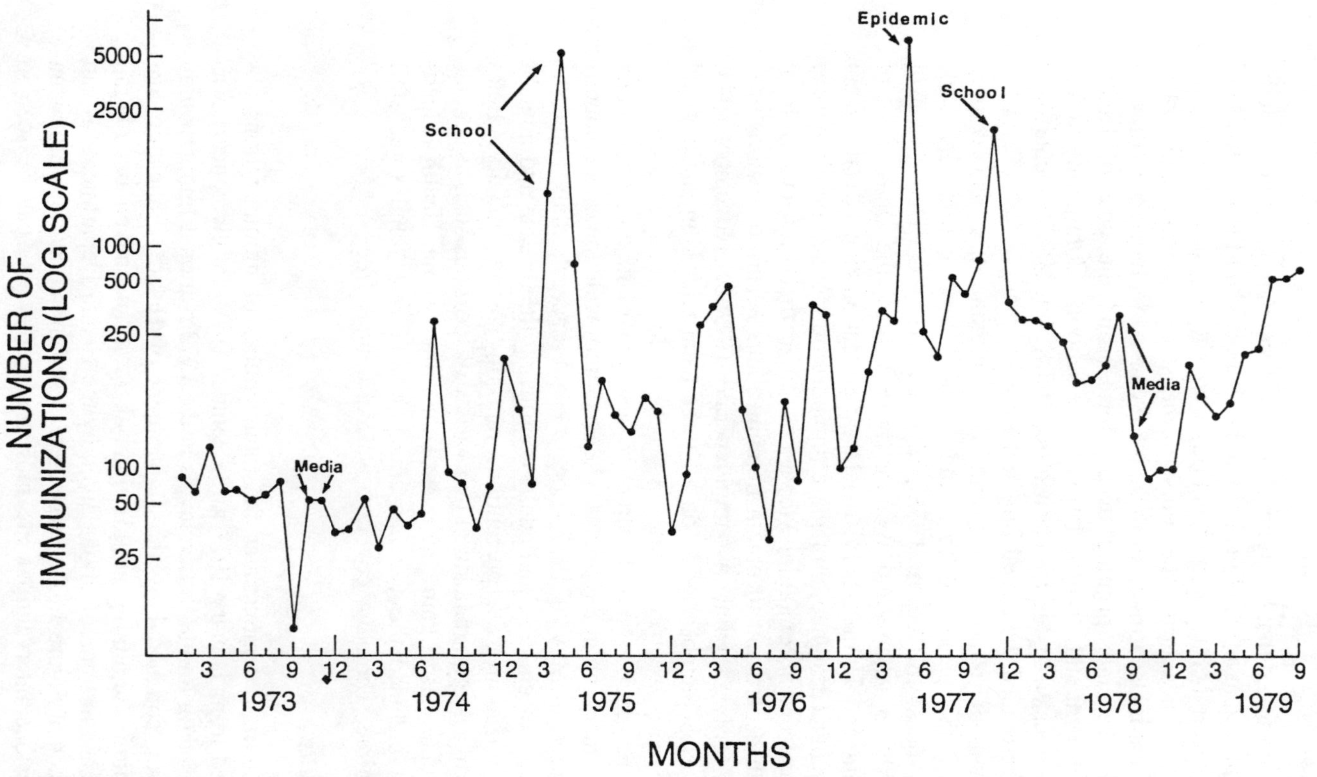

FIGURE 1. Log scale number of immunizations obtained from the Boone County-Columbia City Health Department from January 1973 to September 1979. Arrows indicate community wide DHEW media based public service announcements (labeled "Media"), milestone school based prompts and clinics (labeled "School"), and a local rubella epidemic advertised in the media and accompanied by special local immunization clinics (labeled "Epidemic").

84

school clinic intervention in March-April 1975—immunizations rose from a previous high of 283 immunizations per month (July, 1974) and an average of around 97 per month in 1974 to a total of 6675 for the months of March and April 1975 combined. Similar striking increases followed the second school intervention in November 1977 when immunizations rose to 2276 for the month. These increases each were seen only during the months of the clinic interventions and then the number of immunizations given fell to just below preclinic levels.

In contrast, the two kinds of community wide interventions produced very differing levels of effectiveness. The DHEW advertisement campaigns in October-November of 1973 and August-September of 1978 resulted in no appreciable increase in immunization levels (respectively 52 and 301 immunizations). However, the measles epidemic and resulting community clinics in May 1977 did result in a very large increase in the number of immunizations obtained (6753 for that month alone).

Discussion

The results of the milestone approach to immunizing school-age children indicate that this method was extremely successful in increasing immunizations in this community. Although these data provide a measure only of immunizations given by the Health Department, they parallel the findings of similar studies with school populations (Vernon et al., 1976). The expense of such a program was relatively low, involving only the time of volunteer mothers and students needed to review school records and send forms home to the parents of underimmunized children. Thus, in terms of the financial cost to the agency, only vaccine and duplication costs were required and the cost benefit ratio was excellent.

Unfortunately, it appears that when few cases of a disease are reported and immunization status in the community is thought to be high, the apparent low community risk results in fewer immunizations spontaneously obtained by parents (e.g., see Figure 1 and Mortimer, 1978). This lowered risk might result in fewer school clinics being held if their occurrence was not closely monitored by the Health Department. One of the necessities of successful milestone prevention is that intervention must occur routinely (Peterson, Hartmann & Gelfand, 1980), and these findings suggest the importance of the routine use of the milestone approach to increase and maintain the level of school children's immunizations.

In spite of the admirable effectiveness and cost-benefit ratio of this approach, it has shortcomings even when applied regularly. It fails to serve the entire population and thus will not decrease the risk of sterility in adult men not immunized for mumps nor alter birth defects which can occur in the offspring of childbearing-age women who are not immunized and who contract a disease while pregnant. It will not serve those in frail health or the elderly who may be particularly susceptible to severe cases of immunizable diseases. In all of these categories, individuals in lower socioeconomic classes are likely to be less compliant to medical regimens (Blackwell, 1973) and underimmunized in comparison to middle class individuals (Imperato et al., 1974). Most importantly, a milestone approach targeted toward school-age children fails to impact on preschool children who are more at risk than are school children for immunizable diseases (Marcuse, 1975), and who are in a critical period for survival from such diseases (Imperato, 1974). These issues will be addressed further in the following study.

The community wide intervention attempted by DHEW advertisement campaigns did not result in an appreciable increase in immunization levels in this study. The cost of such a program to the community was extremely low since, during the time of this study, the media were required by law to donate space for public service announcements and the announcements themselves were prepared by DHEW. However, at least in the present study, the low cost was matched by a very low benefit. Again, it should be noted that these data measure only those persons immunized by the Health Department. Anecdotal information from three local private practice pediatricians suggested that the DHEW campaigns did not result in an appreciable increase in immunization from this source either, although numerical data are not available to rule out such a result. However, the ad campaigns did specifically mention seeking out immunizations at the local Health Department, and the lack of impact of this intervention is very similar to that reported for other educative techniques (e.g., Imperato et al., 1974). Perhaps the greatest danger of such techniques is the complacency which may result from organizing a campaign, with the accompanying feeling that "something is being done" and "action has been taken," regardless of the actual level of success (Bergman, 1979). The continued use of such campaigns in the absence of data regarding their effectiveness might even prevent more effective interventions from being funded.

The other community wide intervention, although extremely effective, presents a different set of problems. The measles epidemic and accompanying community clinics resulted in large increases in obtained immunizations. In fact, some researchers have speculated that this is the most common way in which the obtaining of immunizations is influenced—when there are few cases of a disease, immunization levels drop until enough individuals are susceptible to the disease, and then the outbreak of the disease causes a resurgence in immunizations until there are again few cases of the disease (Peterson & Butler, 1979). While relatively effective and inexpensive (in terms of immediate financial, not human costs), this method necessitates the risk of the disease imposed on many and the actual occurrence of the disease in at least a few members of the community. The actual long range cost of epidemics will be dependent on the number of people contracting the disease, the severity of their illness, and the likelihood that they or their children will experience handicaps in the future because of the disease.

These data were from retrospective chart audits and thus it is not possible to rule out increased accuracy in record keeping as a contributing factor in the increase in immunizations over the period of years involved in the study. However, this explanation is viewed by the Health Department officials as unlikely since early records are believed to be quite accurate. In any case, record keeping accuracy would not seem to account for the large impact of clinic interventions or the poor impact of media interventions.

It should be noted that the present conclusions are limited to the specific interventions presented in this study; they do not have relevance for the use of milestone or community wide approaches in general. Some community wide approaches involving media based campaigns, for example, have been quite successful (e.g., de la Burde & Reames, 1973, decreasing ingestion of lead; or Coates & Perry, 1981, Stanford Five City Multifactor Risk Reduction Program), while others have had little impact (Pless, 1978, increasing child safety restraints; Mackay & Rothman, 1982, burn prevention). In general, the more active and costly the behavior requested of the viewer, the less likely the success of the intervention (Baker, 1980). For example, the most effective interventions for child injury prevention have involved one-time legislated mandates for safer products, such as cribs with slats designed to prevent infant strangulation. One time consumer changes, such as setting water thermostats back, are also successful. Daily habit changes such as turning pot handles in while cooking or providing continuous supervision of children during baths are much more difficult to institute, because they are effortful, requiring the agent to remember and reimplement the change repeatedly.

The present findings are meaningful insofar as they describe typical interventions for elevating children's immunization levels. In fact, all of the interventions described here are routinely used in this area and thus these data may suggest specific applications of milestone and high risk group methods for future interventions toward increasing immunizations. Future research could profit from the use of the records of private practice pediatricians, in addition to data from local health agencies, to demonstrate the generality of the present milestone and community wide intervention methods, to truly assess both the costs and the extended benefits of these programs.

The second study outlines an individually oriented program which, like the milestone and community wide methods, attempted to keep costs low and the likelihood of implementation high, while utilizing Bloom's (1968) third method of intervention—targeting individual children who were at high risk. There are many factors which might be selected as identifying risk. Past research has suggested that low socioeconomic preschoolers are most at risk for the immunizable diseases (Marcuse, 1975). Since data from the above described clinics held during the measles epidemic suggested that preschoolers were underserved, and since the milestone approach previously described ruled out preschool children, individual low socioeconomic status preschool children previously served by the Health Department were selected as being at high risk.

STUDY 2

Method

Subjects

A group of 144 underimmunized preschool children was randomly selected from the files of children who had been seen at least once by the Boone County-Columbia City Health Department. The chart audit to identify this group took a volunteer approximately 9 hours to complete. The cost to the Health Department was minimal. The children had in the past been brought in by their parents directly or had been referred by private practice pediatricians or social workers. Prior to their being treated at the Health Department, these children had been determined by health department staff to be from economically underprivileged families who could not rely on another health care agent and they were located within easy traveling distance from the Health Department. In each case the child and the child's family had been seen by the Health Department at least once.

Procedure

A plan similar to that used in the school clinic intervention described in Study 1 was utilized, including prompts to parents, appointment arranging, and a free immunization clinic. When possible, parents were contacted by phone and informed of their child's need for immunization. For all parents with telephone listings, at least five calls were attempted, with at least one call in the morning, afternoon, and evening. For parents without telephone numbers listed in the medical chart, the telephone company was contacted to see if that family had a listing. When parents could not be contacted by telephone, they were sent a letter outlining their child's immunization history and current need for immunization. In both telephone interviews and letters, parents were told of the free clinic and were informed that if they could not come to the free clinic on the dates specified, they could call a given number to arrange another appointment. Both forms of contact suggested that if transportation was a problem, it could be arranged. Parents were also asked to note if their child had received immunization else-where. Those parents receiving letters also received a stamped, addressed postcard to return to the Health Department with desig-nated spaces to update the child's immunization record. The cost to the Health Department included postage and paper materials. Two volunteers completed the calls and letters in approximately 20 hours.

Results

Of the 144 families of children whose files were selected, 23 had no current address or phone number and could not be contacted. Sixty-seven had an address but no phone number; letters were sent to these families. Twenty-five letters were returned with no forwarding address. None of the families to whom letters were sent attended the clinic or called for another appointment, and none returned the postcard indicating that immunization had been received elsewhere.

The remaining 54 families who had operating telephone numbers were repeatedly called as indicated above. Of these, 22 families who could not be reached by phone received letters. Thirty-two parents were reached by telephone; three refused (no reason given) to bring their child in for immunization, six noted that they had already obtained the necessary immunizations elsewhere, and the remaining 23 agreed to come to the immunization clinic. Only 14 of these families actually brought the preschooler to the Health Department for immunizations.

Discussion

The results of this attempt at high risk prevention can be viewed from two differing perspectives. First, the portion of the program involving telephone contact could be viewed as moderately successful, with 19% of those contacted reporting that their preschool child was already fully immunized and with 44% of the families contacted actually bringing their child in for immunization. The cost for this portion of the program was relatively low (just the chart audit time and the time for the telephone interviews, both accomplished by volunteers). These results compare favorably to other programs with very similar sample sizes aimed at high risk preschool children. For example, Minear and Guyer (1979) report on a program which utilized both prompts and home visits by a nurse and resulted in only 32% improvement at a cost of $2,460.

However, there is another equally realistic way of interpreting these data. While an acceptable number of those parents who could be contacted by telephone did bring their child in for immunization, an equally large proportion of those reached by telephone did not. In addition, none of those parents receiving letters rather than telephone contact took advantage of the free clinic; other investigators report similar lack of success with written prompts alone (e.g., Yokley et al., 1980). Finally, a number of these parents with high risk preschoolers had moved, leaving no forwarding address. If the entire sample is considered, only 10% of the preschoolers at risk were immunized due to this program.

There is an undeniable but naturally occurring selection bias in the present study. Families with a consistent address who have a telephone listing may be socially and economically more stable than the other families in the study. While the preschoolers in these families were underimmunized, it seems likely that the families without a telephone who could not be contacted or contacted by letter only were economically more underprivileged and more underserved in terms of medical care than families contacted by phone. Further, this sample was drawn from children already in contact with the Health Department. There is undoubtedly a group of lower socioeconomic status children who have had no medical care, and these children are likely to be even more underimmunized.

The present data do provide a realistic appraisal of what can actually be done in terms of effective immunization in this select high risk group. In general, when no telephone or address is present, there is no economical way of contacting the family. When an address but no telephone is present, either a home visit or a letter appear to be the only possible vehicles. Since home visits for purely preventive purposes are viewed as unacceptably expensive by many (e.g., Bergman, 1979), a letter would seem to be the only recourse. However, since written prompts (which in this case contained the same information as the effective verbal prompts) may not be effective, the most efficient expenditure of time using prompts alone may be to contact only families of high risk children who can be reached by phone. Alternatively, offering monetary rewards for obtaining immunizations (Yokley et al., 1980) or offering special clinics aimed at reducing the inconvenience of obtaining immunizations (perhaps at shopping centers or supermarkets located in low socioeconomic status neighborhoods) may be demonstrated to be even more effective. However, the extra cost and effort of such programs may result in a very low level of actual implementation.

GENERAL DISCUSSION

Bloom (1968) describes three kinds of intervention strategies for effecting primary prevention. Recent research on improving immunization status has focused, in most cases, on high risk group intervention and few if any studies have explored all three methods of intervention within the same community. The present studies offer information concerning the influence of the most commonly

employed milestone, community wide and high risk group interventions on immunization obtaining in a single community agency.
Because of methodological restrictions such as the lack of comparative data from private practice physicians, the generalization of
these data to those individuals obtaining immunization from their
own physicians cannot be assumed. However, in each intervention
the data which are reported are similar to data reported in past
studies. For the most part, the strength of these data is in their
illustration of the potential positive and negative aspects of three
particular forms of intervention for this single community.

Briefly, the milestone program of school clinics described in the
present report was offered at a low cost and it was apparently very
effective. However, to continue to protect children, the intervention
must be administered routinely, and this is often not done (Peterson
& Butler, 1979). Furthermore, many groups requiring immunization were not contacted with a school-age milestone approach. The
community wide media campaigns were offered at a relatively low
cost (although it could be argued that the public service broadcast
time could be used in a more profitable way), but they did not seem
to result in an appreciable increase in immunization. Epidemics and
related clinics reported by the media also had a low immediate cost
and a high rate of effectiveness, but the long term costs may be
prohibitive. Epidemics are also not under the control of those
wishing to plan interventions. Finally, the high risk intervention was
the most costly of the methods described (although the costs were
minor, involving only postage and cost of the forms which were
mailed). This intervention was moderately effective but only with
the telephone subsample of the high risk group. This intervention
also examined only one of the many groups which might be
considered to be at risk for immunizable diseases. Issues of
cost-effectiveness in the end must contain all aspects of cost,
including staff time, and all aspects of effectiveness, including the
ultimate level of protection established within children of differing
developmental levels.

Again, it must be acknowledged that these data do not provide
general conclusions on the efficacy of optimal milestone, community wide, or high risk research, nor do they provide an effective
comparison of these methods in general. A comparison would
require similar content and timing of methods not present in these
studies. Further, each of these methods could undoubtedly be
improved, so the present comparisons could not be said to be

between the optimal examples of each technique, although it seems legitimate to regard each as somewhat effective.

The methods which were maximally effective may have had two features in common which have been described as relevant to preventive health programs (Becker, Haefner, Kasi, Kirschy, Maiman & Rosenstock, 1977). These features include a perceived threat (susceptibility to a currently present disease in the measles epidemic intervention and the legal necessity of immunizing their child in the school clinic intervention), and a perceived reduction in the cost of obtaining preventive care (in both of the successful interventions outlined in Study 1, special clinics reduced the cost of obtaining immunization by offering free immunizations at easily located centers). Future work in improving immunization levels might consider the applicability of these two factors to the less successful methods of intervention here, especially the focus on high risk groups, to see if their manipulation might influence immunization obtaining. For example, if the risk of disease could be made more clear or enrollment in day care or Head Start experiences could be linked to immunization, improvement in immunization levels might result. Similarly, if obtaining immunization could be streamlined by daycare, church or community center clinics, immunizations might be increased. Most importantly, future research must consider the goals and values of the community. In addition, each of the interventions has both explicit costs (such as transportation costs, and costs for postage) and implicit costs (such as the loss of personal freedom when individuals are legally required to be immunized), as well as explicit benefits (such as increases in immunization status) and implicit benefits (such as being better informed about health care). The exact financial costs of the interventions have not been considered here, nor have multiple other factors, such as staff and volunteer time and effort which might be directed elsewhere but for which no direct pricing exists. Also, implicit costs and benefits (e.g., the implicit benefit of establishing a health care routine and of knowing that the child is protected) may be as important as explicit costs and benefits (e.g., actual protection from disease). Furthermore, different sectors of the population are affected dissimilarly, in terms of costs and benefits, by the differing interventions. The elderly who are at high risk for illness are not impacted by school clinics and immunization in low SES community centers will not influence underimmunized middle class children. Thus, the methods used in further attempts to improve community compliance to immunization regimens should be selected with full awareness of the possible choices, the chance for full implementation of the choices, and the costs and benefits of those choices for members of the immediate community.

REFERENCES

Baker, S. P. (1980). Prevention of childhood injuries. *Medical Journal of Australia, 1*, 466-470.

Barkin, S. Z., Barkin, R. M. & Roth, M. L. (1977). Immunization status: A parameter of patient compliance. *Clinical Pediatrics, 16*, 840-842.

Becker, M. H., Haefner, D. P., Kasi, S. V., Kirschy, J. P., Maiman, L. A. & Rosenstock, I. M. (1977). Selected psychosocial models and correlates of individual health-related behaviors. *Medical Care, 15*, 27-46.

Bergman, A. B. (1979). Califano's body counts. *Pediatrics, 63*, 27-46.

Blackwell, B. (1973). Patient compliance. *New England Journal of Medicine, 289*, 249.

Bloom, B. L. (1968). The evaluation of primary prevention programs. In L. M. Roberts, N. S. Greenfield & M. H. Miller (eds.), *Comprehensive mental health: The challenge of evaluation.* Madison: University of Wisconsin Press.

Coates, T. J. & Perry, C. (1981). Multifactor risk reduction with children and adolescents taking care of the heart in behavior group therapy. In D. Upper & S. Ross (eds.), *Behavior group therapy: An annual review.* Champaign, IL: Research Press.

de la Burde, B. & Reames, B. (1973). Prevention of pica, the major cause of lead poisoning in children. *American Journal of Public Health, 6*, 737-743.

Imperato, P. J. (1974). The present status of diphtheria in New York City. *Bulletin of the New York Academy of Medicine, 50*, 763-776.

Imperato, P. J., Pincus, L., Hwa, C. L. & Chaves, A. D. (1974). The control of measles in New York City. *Bulletin of the New York Academy of Medicine, 50*, 602-619.

Krugman, S. & Katz, S. L. (1977). Childhood immunization procedures. *Journal of the American Medical Association, 321*, 2228-2230.

Mackay, A. M. & Rothman, K. J. (1982). The incidence and severity of burn injuries following Project Burn Prevention. *American Journal of Public Health, 72*, 248-252.

Marcuse, E. K. (1975). Immunization: An embarrassing failure. *Pediatrics, 56*, 493-494.

Minear, R. E. & Guyer, B. (1979). Assessing immunization services at a neighborhood health center. *Pediatrics, 63*, 416-419.

Mortimer, E. A. (1978). Immunization against infectious disease. *Science, 200*, 902-907.

Peterson, L. & Butler, R. (1979). *A behavioral model of the analysis of childhood immunizations.* Paper presented at the meeting of the Association for Behavior Analysis, Dearborn, Michigan.

Peterson, L., Hartmann, D. R. & Gelfand, D. M. (1980). Prevention of child behavior disorders: A lifestyle change for child psychologists. In P. O. Davidson & S. M. Davidson (eds.), *Behavioral medicine: Changing health lifestyles.* New York: Brunner/Mazel.

Peterson, L. & Mori, L. (1985). Prevention of child injury: An overview of targets, methods, and tactics for psychologists. *Journal of Consulting and Clinical Psychology, 53*, 586-595.

Peterson, L. & Ridley-Johnson, R. (1983). Prevention of disorders in children. In C. E. Walker & M. C. Roberts (eds.), *Handbook of clinical child psychology.* New York: John-Wiley.

Pless, I. B. (1978). Accident prevention and health education: Back to the drawing board? *Pediatrics, 62*, 431-435.

Roberts, M. C., Elkins, P. D. & Royal, G. P. (1984). Psychological applications to the prevention of accidents and illness. In M. C. Roberts & L. Peterson (eds.), *Prevention of problems in childhood: Psychological research and applications*. New York: Wiley-Interscience.

Rossi, J., Freeman, S. & Wright, A. (1979). *Evaluation: A systematic approach*. Beverly Hills: Sage Publications.

Vernon, T. M., Connor, J. S., Shaw, B. S., Lampe, J. M. & Doster, M. E. (1976). An evaluation of three techniques for improving immunization levels in elementary schools. *American Journal of Public Health, 66*, 457-460.

Yokley, J. M., Glenwick, D. W., Hedrick, T. E. & Page, N. D. (1980). *Increasing the immunization of high risk preschoolers: An evaluation of applied community interventions*. Paper presented at the meeting of the Association for Advancement of Behavior Therapy, New York.

The Preventive Role
of Breastfeeding

Derrick B. Jelliffe
E. F. Patrice Jelliffe
University of California

SUMMARY. The preventive role of breastfeeding is examined in the context of evidence from comparative lactation and in light of recent scientific knowledge. Preventive advantages are discussed in relation to nutrition, infections, allergy, emotional development, contraception and economics and food production. It is concluded that breastfeeding has a considerable preventive role in both technically less and more developed countries, but that the main aspects of such prevention vary considerably with circumstances and risks.

Research of recent years has illustrated ever more clearly the great and important differences arising from the process of breastfeeding human milk and that of bottle-feeding, using cow's milk-based formulas. The preventive benefits of breastfeeding can best be appreciated if it is viewed in the context of recent work on comparative lactation and in relation to advances in scientific knowledge. This paper summarizes such developments and their significance for prevention.

COMPARATIVE LACTATION

Adaptive Suckling

Over eons, each mammal species has evolved a highly specific and complex composition of maternal milk and a delivery process appropriate for the species' particular way of life; these provide protective mechanisms such as a generalized anti-infective effect and influence birth spacing. For example, the female dolphin

---

Reprints may be obtained from Derrick B. Jelliffe, School of Public Health, University of California, Los Angeles, CA 90024.

97

secretes milk which is very rich in calories and fat and has a very powerful milk-ejection reflex. Adaptive suckling by the young dolphin takes the form of a rapid pumping for "cream" because of its high calorie needs and because it can hold its breath for only a limited period of time.

Such a developmental adaptation of suckling behavior has occurred over lengthy periods of time—1 or 2 million years in the case of *Homo erectus*. These evolutionary changes are teleonomic—that is, they are the result of natural selection ensuring the optimum growth and protection of vulnerable infants and the survival of the particular species.

Biological Infant Feeding

To understand the complexity and adaptations of human milk and human breastfeeding, it is helpful to consider this process as "biological infant feeding." Such a concept differs from the customary, more restricted view of infant feeding in western countries, where it is often considered solely as a mathematical process for dietary refuelling. Information to guide rational infant feeding practices should be obtained from a variety of sources— from fellow, nonhuman mammals, from present-day traditional societies, from past practices in the West, and from metabolic data, which are, however, increasingly recognized as imperfect, variable and subject to many subtle, newly identified adaptations. Such a wider view of infant feeding considers the process not only as one for the supply of nutrients but also as having effects on mother-child interaction, protection against infection, child spacing, economics and food supply.

RECENT SCIENTIFIC KNOWLEDGE

In the last decade, a flood of new knowledge has become available as the unique significance of human milk and breastfeeding has become increasingly apparent (Jelliffe & Jelliffe, 1978; Lawrence, 1981). This includes information on the specific biochemical composition of human milk, its anti-infective, anti-allergenic properties, contraceptive effects and the implications for economics and food production (see Table 1 which is adapted from Jelliffe & Jelliffe, 1984).

Table 1

Recently Recognized Preventive Attributes of Human Milk and Breastfeeding

Attribute	Preventive Effect
Biochemical Composition	
Zinc-binding compound	Bioavailability (leads to improved absorption of zinc)
Breast milk lipase (enzyme)	Rapid digestion of fat
High content of taurine (amino acid negligible in cow's milk)	Optimal supply for development of retina and parts of brain
Hormones, enzymes, and numerous growth modulators	Probable decreasing need for certain nutrients and growth stimulation of specific tissues
Anti-Infective Properties	
Clean with no opportunity for bacterial multiplication	
Live white cells present and wide range of protective substances	Protection against bacterial and viral intestinal infections
Anti-parasitic substances	Lethal to Giardia lamblia and Entamoeba histolytica
Anti-Allergenic Effects	
Presence of secretory IgA (antibody)	Limits absorption of foreign protein
Absence of large amounts of cow's milk protein	Protection against infantile cow's milk protein allergy
Contraception	
Hormonal secretion, prolactin, etc., from frequent feeding	Delays menstruation and enhances biological child spacing
Economics and Food Production	
Major national resource	Important in achieving food self-sufficiency and saving currency

Specific Biochemical Composition

Four particular substances and their effects may be noted which have particular protective, preventive roles (Table 1). Of particular species-specific interest are the recently recognized "growth modulators," whose hormone-like role in stimulating the growth of specific tissues, including the central nervous system and cells of the intestine, is only beginning to be studied and understood (Ebrahim, 1982).

Anti-Infective Properties

Until recently, it was believed that the protective effect of human milk against some infections, notably diarrhea, occurs because it is clean and relatively uncontaminated. This is true, but recent studies have shown that human milk also contains large numbers of white cells and an increasingly recognized range of protective substances (Table 1) (Wilkinson, 1981).

In addition, it has been shown that the organisms with which the mother comes into contact are countered by specific protective substances which are present in her milk. One way in which this occurs is via the so-called "gut-mammary axis." This means that the mother and baby have a close, two-way interaction as regards bacterial flora. Microorganisms entering the mother's alimentary canal lead to increases in specific protective substances in her milk. This protection mediates against the infant, in turn, picking up the harmful bacteria.

The particular preventive value of colostrum—the yellowish first secretion after birth—was greatly under-emphasized until recently. It was thought that this substance was of little importance, only filling a gap until the mature milk became available. It is now recognized that colostrum is not only rich in protective substances but also contains concentrated doses of certain nutrients, notably vitamins A and E and zinc (Chappell, Francis & Clandinin, 1985).

The cellular composition of human milk has long been recognized scientifically. Biologically, breast milk is a complex fluid; even in prescientific societies, it is often referred to as "white blood." White cells in colostrum and human milk are present in numbers similar to those in the blood. Their effect is not only on the infant but on the mother as well, protecting her against ascending infections that might occur in the milk ducts of the breasts. In addition to direct action, such as engulfing any bacteria present, some milk cells secrete anti-infective substances, including an anti-viral substance—interferon. This is especially important as viruses have become increasingly recognized as a common cause of diarrhea.

The situation with regard to protection against diarrheal disease is highly relevant to this discussion. Newborn infants are especially protected against it by breast milk, and thus diarrhea in the newborn can be regarded as a "colostrum deprivation syndrome." The preventive effect is also very important later in early infancy (from 1 to 6/9 months). As other foods are introduced into the diet during the period of weaning, human milk forms a lesser part of the diet, and its protective effects diminish. Of course, the significance and degree of the anti-diarrheal effects of breast milk varies with the local risks—particularly with respect to environmental hygiene practices, which are themselves dependent on levels of education and economics. The protective benefits of breast milk in a refugee camp, or in a tropical slum, are obviously greater than those in a well-to-do, middle class suburb. To state it differently: the anti-infective effect of human milk is universal but is less obviously important and needed when the risks to infant health are less.

Anti-Allergenic Effects

Ingestion of cow's milk protein has been found to be the commonest cause of food allergy in human infants. Careful studies in some industrial countries have shown that about one percent of bottle-fed babies are so affected (Gruskany, 1982).

The cause of this allergy is simple. Large amounts of foreign proteins are ingested at a time when the infant's intestinal wall is relatively "open" to their absorption from cow's milk formulas. By contrast, human milk contains specific substances that block such absorption. Breastfeeding (and the avoidance of the introduction of semisolids until 4-6 months of age) provides the best prevention against food allergies due to cow's milk protein in infancy, especially in families that have an allergic history or allergic predisposition.

Emotional Benefits

In nonhuman mammals, it has been recognized that bonding between mother and baby occurs at a specific time, resulting from, and leading to, a special pattern of mother-newborn behavior. Recent investigations have also shown that a similar pattern occurs in humans, and that early mother-neonate contact facilitates such bonding to produce a harmonious relationship between mother and baby, as well as to facilitate breastfeeding (Klaus & Kennell, 1983). This bonding process occurs most easily in the immediate postpartum period, and it is expedited by close contact between mother and baby immediately after delivery. The relationship between bonding and breastfeeding has not been clearly established so it has not been included in Table 1.

Contraception

Until very recently, scientific medicine considered the idea that breastfeeding had a child spacing effect as an old wives' tale. This misconception was understandable, as it is clear that pregnancy occurs in some women who are still breastfeeding. Recent endocrinological and epidemiological research has shown, however, that the child spacing effect of breastfeeding is "dose-dependent"— that is, the more the infant sucks, the more the pituitary hormone, prolactin, is produced in the mother. Prolactin effectively delays menstruation and ovulation (Delvoye & Robyn, 1980).

That this occurs in humans is not surprising. All other mammals have appropriate natural methods of spacing their offspring. For many species, this is achieved by having periods of estrus, or mating seasons. In humans, mating is year-round, and natural child spacing is aided by the endocrinological effects of the infant's frequent suckling. Such a child spacing effect can be prolonged. For example, in some communities in Africa, where breastfeeding is frequent and prolonged, and where other foods are not introduced early, the period between one pregnancy and the next can be as much as four years. Conversely, if the amount of infant suckling is restricted, with limited breastfeedings during the day and the use of other foods which reduce the infant's appetite and sucking vigor, the effectiveness of this natural method of child spacing is decreased (Huntington & Hostetler, 1970; Short, 1984).

Economics and Food Production

With the current world economic and food distribution situation, the financial problem represented by bottle-feeding needs emphasis. This can be viewed at the level of individual families; in developing countries, purchase of sufficient formula may require up to 60-80% of a family's basic income. Similar, but less dramatic considerations must prevail in disadvantaged communities everywhere, including the United States.

Even more significant is the fact that breast milk constitutes a major societal resource, both economic and agronomic. It has been calculated, for example, that if all women in Indonesia were to cease breastfeeding, an annual expenditure of approximately 52 million dollars would be required to purchase adequate formula supplies, to pay for hospital care for children with diarrheal disease, and to increase family planning services (Rohde, 1982).

CONCLUSION

From the above discussion, it can be appreciated that some harmful effects of artificial feeding with cow's milk-based formulas are universal. In families in disadvantaged circumstances in both industrialized and developing countries, bottle-feeding is likely to result in diarrheal disease and severe malnutrition, with often fatal results (Kanaaneh, 1972). To be able to bottle-feed regularly, three things are required—enough money to purchase appropriate amounts of formula, reasonable home hygiene (including a safe water supply) and sufficient parental education so that the formula is prepared correctly.

However, even in well-to-do families living in superior environments, the risks of bottle-feeding with cow's milk-based formulas are considerable. Investigators have shown significant differences in the frequency of episodes of infection occurring in breastfed and bottle-fed babies in such circumstances (Cunningham, 1981). Even more striking is the incidence of infantile allergies to cow's milk protein. In many parts of the world, such as Indonesia, cow's milk protein allergy has been reported by experienced pediatricians in communities when babies move from breast to bottle-feeding.

In addition, the bottle-fed baby experiences a different form of mother-to-baby interaction, with different emotional consequences. The infant who is lovingly bottle-fed does *not* have the same psychological experience as does the breastfed one. The physiological stimuli are different for mother and child. The production and influence of maternal hormones occurs distinctively in the breastfeeding mother and is absent for the mother who is physically distant from thc infant, providing food through a glass or plastic bottle and rubber nipple. Some investigators believe that these effects carry over into the psychological development of the child and to later parent-child relationships (Klaus & Kennell, 1983).

Preventive Effects of Breastfeeding

Table 2 illustrates the relative advantages of breastfeeding for *both* mother and infant in developing and developed countries. Clearly, these benefits and deficits vary; from poor communities, where there is inadequate home hygiene, minimal financial re-

Table 2

Major Preventive Effects of Breastfeeding in Developed Countries (DC) and Less Developed Countries (LDC)

Effects On:	Infant		Mother	
	DC	LDC	DC	LDC
Human Milk				
Nutritional	++	+++		
Anti-infective	++	+++		
Anti-allergic	+++	?		
Economics			+	+++
Breastfeeding Process				
Child spacing		++	+	+++
Bonding	+++	+++	+++	+++
Hormonal effect on uterine			+	+++

Note. + = small effect; ++ = moderate effect; +++ = major effect.

sources, and little parental education, to societies where most women are educated, home hygiene is good and families have sufficient income to purchase adequate supplies of formula.

The relative benefits to infant and mother can be compared in so-called developed (DC) and less developed (LDC) countries (Table 2). The physiological effects of breastfeeding on the mother's uterus is particularly important in areas where maternal anemia during pregnancy is common. Rapid uterine contraction after delivery can inhibit maternal bleeding; this process is speeded-up by certain hormones, especially oxytocin, which are secreted by the breastfeeding woman.

If one looks only at the *nutritional* role of breastfeeding in developing countries, it primarily accomplishes the prevention of one severe form of malnutrition—marasmus (and associated infective diarrhea) in infancy (Jelliffe, Symonds & Jelliffe, 1960). However, its secondary *partial* role in preventing malnutrition in the second year of life is sometimes not recognized. In fact, human milk is *the* food to start with for newborns; after 4-6 months it remains a small, but important, nutritional supplement for growing, older infants.

Recent studies have also confirmed that the anti-infective properties of breast milk (including protection against diarrheal disease), are significant in middle class communities in industrialized countries, especially with respect to the incidence of episodes of infection (Cunningham, 1980). Cunningham has demonstrated this effect in his investigations in New York State (Table 3); there are similar findings from literature from other developed countries (Cunningham, 1981).

In considering the advantages of human milk and breastfeeding as compared with bottle-feeding, one has to take an unfragmented or holistic view. The infant, the family and the community's welfare must be considered in light of the nutritional, emotional, anti-infective, economic and contraceptive effects of breastfeeding.

Public Health Implications

The public health concerns, and the implications of the availability or unavailability of human milk are extensive and increasing but often under-appreciated. These problems and concerns differ in resource-poor and resource-rich countries. In less technically developed, resource-poor countries, Bengoa (1974) has estimated that

Table 3

Number of Episodes per 1,000 Patient-Weeks of Significant Illness According
to Feeding Mode at Onset of Illness in Cooperstown, New York

Illness	Breast-Fed Infants	Bottle-Fed Infants
Otitis media	3.7	9.1
Lower respiratory tract infection	1.1	5.6
Diarrhea, vomiting	3.5	6.9
Hospital admissions	1.0	3.0
Total episodes of illness	8.2	21.1

Note. From Cunningham, 1981.

there are 9.4 million annual cases of severe protein-calorie malnutrition in infants and young children. Assuming conservatively that half of these have marasmus related to bottle-feeding or inadequate lactation, 4.7 million children could be protected wholly or in part by breastfeeding by adequately-nourished mothers.

Because of inadequate data, the number of children with diarrhea associated with bottle-feeding in such countries is difficult to calculate. However, the World Health Organization's surveys show that the condition is very common. If a somewhat higher prevalence figure than for marasmus is projected (5.3 million), partial or complete protection of some 10 million infants annually may be attainable by extended breastfeeding. With an average 30 percent mortality of young sufferers from diarrhea, this would mean 3 million lives could be saved and, postulating an arbitrary figure of $100 per child for treatment, a yearly expenditure of 1 billion dollars avoided.

In the technically more developed and resource-rich countries of the world, more than 11 million births occur annually, and the preventive effects of extending breastfeeding in these societies could also be highly significant. If cow's milk allergy occurs in 1 percent of newborns, the avoidance of cow's milk in the early months of life by breastfeeding could prevent some 100,000 new cases of infantile cow's milk allergy *each* year.

From a family planning perspective, a recent study has estimated that breastfeeding provides 35 million couple-years' protection annually (Rosa, 1976). The increase and improvement of lactation in less developed countries could increase this total significantly. Conversely, declines in breastfeeding would lead to a loss of child spacing protection, an increase in birth rates, and the need for funds and facilities to increase family planning services.

In economic terms, Berg (1973) has calculated that if 20 percent of mothers living in urban areas in all developing countries do not breastfeed, this results in a direct loss of $365 million per year in those nations. In theory, this sum must be at least doubled, as it has to be matched by a similar expense for purchasing breast-milk substitutes, and for financing *additional* maternal and child health services, including family planning.

The harmful consequences of bottle-feeding instead of breast-feeding are widespread, of very large dimensions, and involve millions of infants throughout the world. In the adaptive maternal and child health services urgently required in all countries, promotion of breastfeeding obviously should play a major role. It is inappropriate and dangerous to continue a double-standard approach to breastfeeding—to believe that it is desirable in "primitive" or developing societies but not necessary or pertinent in advanced ones. In fact, its preventive importance is universal.

REFERENCES

Bengoa, J. M. (1974). The problem of undernutrition. *WHO Chronicle, 28*, 3-8.
Berg, A. (1973). *The nutrition factor*. Washington: Brookings Institution.
Chappell, J. E., Francis, T. & Clandinin, M. T. (1985). Vitamin A and E content of human milk at early stages of lactation. *Early Human Development, 11*, 157-161.
Cunningham, A. (1981). Breast-feeding and morbidity in industrialized countries. *Advances in International Maternal and Child Health, 1*, 128-168.
Delvoye, P. & Robyn, C. (1981). Prolactin and post partum amenonlioes. *Journal of Tropical Pediatrics, 26*, 184-189.
Ebrahim, G. J. (1982). Human breast milk: A mediator of biological functions. *Journal of Tropical Pediatrics, 28*, ii-iii.
Gruskay, F. L. (1982). Comparison of breast, cow and soy feedings in the prevention of the onset of allergic disease: 15 year prospective study. *Clinical Pediatrics, 21*, 486-491.
Huntington, G. & Hostekler, J. (1970). A note on nursing practices in an American isolate with a high birth rate. *Population Studies, 24*, 321-330.
Jelliffe, D. B. & Jelliffe, E. F. P. (1978). *Human milk in the modern world*. Oxford: Oxford University Press.

Jelliffe, D. B. & Jelliffe, E. F. P. (1984). Breast-milk policy. *World Health Forum, 5*, 37-38.

Jelliffe, D. B., Symonds, B. E. R. & Jelliffe, E. F. P. (1960). The pattern of malnutrition in southern Trinidad. *Journal of Pediatrics, 57*, 922-926.

Kanaaneh, H. (1972). The relationship of bottle feeding to malnutrition and gastroenteritis in a pre-industrial setting. *Journal of Tropical Pediatrics, 18*, 302-306.

Klaus, M. & Kennell, J. (1983). Parent-infant bonding: Setting the record straight. *Journal of Pediatrics, 102*, 575-579.

Lawrence, R. A. (1981). *Breastfeeding: A guide for the medical profession*. St. Louis: Mosby.

Rohde, J. E. (1982). Mother's milk and the Indonesian economy. *Journal of Tropical Pediatrics, 28*, 166-169.

Rosa, F. W. (1974). Breast feeding and family planning. *Journal of Tropical Pediatrics, 20*, 1-2.

Short, R. V. (1984). Breastfeeding. *Scientific American, 250*, 35-39.

Wilkinson, A. W. (ed.) (1981). *The immunology of infant feeding*. New York: Plenum.

Synergy and Healing:
A Perspective
on Western Health Care

Richard Katz
University of Alaska-Fairbanks
Harvard University

Niti Seth
Harvard University

SUMMARY. There is a crisis in health care resulting from the scarcity of resources and the inequitable distribution of those resources toward those most able to pay. Two paradigms for the generation and distribution of resources are discussed. The scarcity paradigm, in which individuals must compete for scarce resources, dominates Western care and expresses and supports that crisis. The synergy paradigm, in which individuals share resources which are renewable and expanding, is rare in the West but could help alleviate that crisis. Three case studies of synergy in Western health care are presented, illustrating the nature and functioning of "synergistic community." Dilemmas remaining in the introduction and maintenance of synergy within Western care are discussed.

A group of health providers from a major university in the United States invited Dr. Fendor, an authority in preventive health care, to spend a day at their university discussing her ideas.[1] Dr. Fendor based her work on a dialogical approach, in the manner of Paulo Freire (1968). Her central tenet was that she was not the expert who possessed special knowledge about health care, but only the initiator of a process of dialogue with her clients, and from that dialogue, clients became empowered and capable of their own preventive efforts. One learned about Dr. Fendor's health care approach by

We wish to thank Karen Davison, Jared A. Hermalin, Kenneth Lappin, Ceasar McDowell, Fernando Mederos, Maureen Reese and, especially, Rob Hess for their thoughtful, generous, and helpful comments on earlier drafts of this paper. Reprints may be obtained from Richard Katz, Department of Behavioral Science, College of Human and Rural Development, Gruening Building, University of Alaska-Fairbanks, Fairbanks, Alaska 99775-1380.

109

engaging in it; knowledge about health care, and health care itself, merged.

Dr. Fendor was a world-renowned authority and the group of health providers who invited her to the university was keenly interested in her work. Moreover, her trips to the states were infrequent and so the occasion of her visit represented a "rare opportunity" for the group. And in that lay the problem.

The group met to plan Dr. Fendor's visit and immediately faced a dilemma. All agreed that the visit represented an important opportunity to learn about health care; they disagreed on how best to accomplish that learning. One faction in the group wanted the visit to be centered around a series of small, intensive seminars, attended by Dr. Fendor, the planning group, and a few more invited health care professionals. They reasoned that Dr. Fendor was uniquely knowledgeable about her approach to health care—she was the valued resource. It was important to maximize direct contact with her, they argued, but since there was only one of her, and many wanted access to her, it was best to keep the sessions small. That would reduce the competition to be with Dr. Fendor, they said.

A second faction wanted the visit to be centered around a series of open meetings in which all those with a sincere interest in Dr. Fendor's ideas would be welcome to attend. This second faction reasoned that Dr. Fendor should be taken at her word; that she was not unique in her health care knowledge, but part of a *process* of care which was initiated by her being in dialogue with others. If dialogue was initiated—and only if it was, did her approach to preventive health care become an actuality—then all participants in the dialogue were of value, and the more who participated the more empowering was the dialogue for more people. The dialogue process itself would become the valued resource, not Dr. Fendor; the valued resource, therefore, was expanding, not limited. Access to dialogue did not depend on direct contact with Dr. Fendor, but on a willingness to engage in dialogue with other participants—a willingness not dependent on possessing expert knowledge.

The second faction carried the day and planned the visit. Just as they hoped for, the resource of preventive health care, expressed in the dialogical process, expanded and was renewed as Dr. Fendor stimulated but then became part of that process. Those attending the day reported being effected in the very ways they were learning to effect others; they felt more empowered to become responsible for their own health care. One participant put it this way:

> It was great to see Dr. Fendor among us. I realized this was not the great woman coming to help the disciples, but all of us gathering to help each other and ourselves. We had today what I always wish I could stimulate in my own work: a community which cared and cared for itself.

The two plans for Dr. Fendor's visit represented two contrasting ways to organize experience and distribute resources, two patterns in which and by which phenomena are related to each other. The experience and pattern of resource distribution planned by the first faction would have illustrated the "scarcity" paradigm; the experience and pattern of resource distribution planned by the second faction—and eventually actualized—illustrated the "synergy" paradigm. "Synergy" and "scarcity" are difficult concepts to describe, but they seem essential to understand if we are to begin meeting the pressing challenges in preventive health care.

In an earlier paper (Katz, 1983/84), we delineated these two paradigms for the generation and distribution of valued resources, one based upon "scarcity," the other on "synergy." Focusing on healing as a valued resource, we suggested that in the West[2] healing typically functions within a scarcity paradigm; healing becomes a scarce resource, requiring competition for access, resulting in inequitable usage. We argued that healing resources belong intrinsically within a synergy paradigm and, therefore, would become renewable and expanding, and accessible equitably throughout the community; the result was called a "synergistic community." The emphasis was on one typical context for this synergistic approach to health: traditional, non-Western societies. The present paper shifts the focus to the West, where synergistic community is less common. We consider how synergy can be a response in the West to the worldwide crisis in health care, where increasing need is not being met by an increase in resources as limited high-cost treatments, which are inequitably distributed, are emphasized more than low-cost and pervasive prevention efforts (World Health Organization, 1976). This paper poses a challenge: how can Western approaches to health and healing move away from the scarcity paradigm to function more within a synergy paradigm, so that healing becomes more of a renewable, expanding resource which is shared on a more equitable basis?

SYNERGY AND SYNERGISTIC COMMUNITY: A REVIEW OF THE CONCEPTS

The concepts of synergy and synergistic community may seem elusive. They describe a special quality, something in the "atmosphere" or "climate" of a group when it is resonating, functioning beyond words. Yet the actual *experience* of synergy and synergistic community, which is the important focus, is palpable, concrete, and easily recognized by those who experience it. Despite the difficulty of defining these concepts, their potential contribution to scarcity-based Western health care justifies our further study of them. We can begin our study by briefly examining how synergy and synergistic community function among the !Kung of the Kalahari Desert, a people who in many ways exemplify these concepts.

It is appropriate to begin with the !Kung, who live primarily as hunter-gatherers (Katz, 1982; Lee, 1979; Marshall, 1976). Though hunting-gathering is rare today, the !Kung are *representative* of what was the universal pattern of human existence for 99% of cultural history. It is generally agreed that the basic dimensions of human nature were forged during that huge span of time (Lee & DeVore, 1968). The !Kung can, therefore, provide fundamental and crucial insights for understanding processes of human adaptation and the structure of social organization. In particular, the !Kung can teach us about fundamental issues in synergy and community and their impact on health care.

The !Kung exemplify synergistic community in various ways. Land—and the water, food, and materials provided thereon—is perhaps their most valued resource. It is utilized in a synergistic manner. Local groups neither maintain exclusive rights to resources nor defend territories; a reciprocal access prevails. Food resources are not accumulated by individuals as the environment itself acts as the storehouse. When brought into camp, food is distributed to all to be consumed. Frequent visiting among groups mitigates the effects of localized food shortages, and when food resources in a particular area become scarce, groups scatter more widely over the environment (Lee, 1979; Marshall, 1976).

Another most valued resource is *n/um* or "spiritual energy"

(Katz, 1982; Marshall, 1969). N/um, representing what is powerful, has primary significance throughout !Kung life. It appears in its most intense form during the healing dance, the primary !Kung ritual. When n/um is "boiling" in the healers, it provides healing to the community which has gathered to create the dance. Healing for the !Kung is an integrating and enhancing force, far more fundamental than simple curing. The dance initiates synergistic community (Katz, 1982).

N/um is renewable, available with each new dance. As it is activated, it expands and becomes accessible to all as all are given healing. Giving healing to one person makes it more likely it will be given to others. "When n/um rises," said one healer, "it spreads among the people like sparks that fly from a strongly stirred fire." The !Kung do not allow n/um to be controlled by a few religious specialists; almost half the adults are healers. N/um is released by the community, and through its healing effects, helps to recreate and renew that community.

Knowledge influenced by n/um partakes of its synergistic quality (Katz, 1981; 1982). Knowing how to activate n/um to produce healing is highly valued; it is knowledge about the culture's deepest mysteries. The community is the repository of knowledge about n/um; as the dance releases that knowledge in individual healers, they share it with the community. Learning to become a healer is a community responsibility. Though students may work with a particular teacher or two, members of the community at large also have important teaching roles during the dance.

Synergy and scarcity represent paradigmatic alternatives, two ends of a continuum which in actual situations exist in some combination (Katz, 1983/84). The scarcity paradigm assumes that valued resources are scarce; their presumed scarcity contributes largely to their being valued. It further assumes that individuals or communities must compete with each other to gain access to these resources, continually struggling to accumulate their own supply as they continually exhaust it, resisting pressures to share, resulting in an inequitable distribution of the resource.

Synergy describes a pattern in and by which phenomena are related to each other (Fuller, 1963; Katz, 1982; Maslow & Honigmann, 1970). A synergistic pattern exists when phenomena are interrelating so that an often unexpectedly bountiful and greater whole is created from disparate, seemingly conflicting parts which are often combined in an apparently illogical manner. In that pattern, phenomena exist in harmony with each other, maximizing each others' potential. Individuals and communities activate resources. They function as guardians, not possessors, of resources and while guided by the motivation of service to others, they allow resources to be shared by all members of the community. Greater amounts of the resource become increasingly available to all so that collaboration rather than competition is encouraged. Paradoxically, the more the resource is utilized, the more there is to be utilized.

"Synergistic community" is a perspective for understanding the functioning of synergy within a community as well as a guideline for increasing that synergy (Katz, 1983/84). Synergistic community is established when members experience an enhancement of consciousness which brings on both a sense of self-embedded-in-community and actions which express that embeddedness (Katz, 1983/84). The enhancement of consciousness need not be radical or intense, often it is a subtle shift in perspective. As boundaries of the self become more permeable to a dimension beyond the self, a transpersonal bonding occurs between people so that individuals activate communal commitments. As persons go beyond individual needs, sharing of resources becomes possible, even predictable. Realizing their deep connectedness, people realize they need not compete for resources, which have become shared and thereby expandable.

We offer our definitions of synergy and synergistic community aware of major limitations. As did James (1936) in his efforts to define noetic experiences, we realize our definitions emphasize the *actual* experience. As did Turner (1969) in his efforts to define the experiences of "liminality" and "communitas," we realize our definitions of synergy depend heavily on knowing what is *not* synergy. Turner relies on our knowledge of structure and structured experience to understand liminality and communitas, which he considers examples of "anti-structure." As did Sarason (1977) in his efforts to define the experience of "psychological sense of community," we realize our definitions depend heavily on the presupposition that those who experience synergy will know it. Yet synergy and synergistic community also differ from these related concepts: while partaking of the more spiritual quality of James' religious experiences, synergy and synergistic community are also more practical, mundane, and concrete; while partaking of the unstructured, "betwixt and between" condition of "liminality" and "communitas," they do not entail a return to structure, even to the status quo; and while partaking of the interpersonal connectedness in the "psychological sense of community," they go beyond the psychological and interpersonal toward a transpersonal bonding.

Our definitions point to the fact that synergistic community is not merely equivalent to "sharing" or "cooperation," or to "good feelings" in a group or community, or a "sense of togetherness." Synergy is not equivalent to "good group process" or to positive communal experiences. Special conditions must prevail for synergy to exist, such as valued resources in the community being *renewable, expanding*, and *accessible to all*. The *paradoxical* and *generative* quality of synergy, in which the more you use a resource, the more it is there to be used, does not, for example, exist in all instances of sharing or group collaboration.

Synergy is an inevitable aspect or phase of community, existing in a dialectical, but non-dualistic relationship with scarcity. Communities which function primarily within the scarcity paradigm require at least brief moments of synergy to hold them together; likewise, communities cannot always function synergistically. Synergistic community refers both to the phase of synergy that is intrinsic to community and to those particular communities in which the balance is toward synergy.

What are the necessary or sufficient factors for the emergence of synergistic community? Are the economics of valued resources being expandable and renewable a sufficient factor? Is the socio-cultural structure of the community that distributes these resources equitably a necessary factor? How powerful a factor is a common mythology or belief system, which makes sharing of valued resources a simple fact of life, or a motivation to share, and a willingness to experience the sense of vulnerability which takes one beyond the individual self and towards transpersonal bonding? Most likely, a combination of factors is necessary. Then we need not rely, for example, on the assumptions of humanistic psychology, such as the good-will or self-actualizing tendency of people. Synergy can result even if people are not especially generous or altruistic but because they participate in a social structure which makes their pursuit of their own best interest simultaneously serve the common good (Katz, 1983/84; Maslow & Honigmann, 1970).

Healing seen as a "transitioning toward balance, meaning, connectedness and wholeness" (Katz, 1982) exemplifies a resource synergistically activated; hence healing is an intrinsically renewable resource. Healing communities can exemplify synergistic community; they are, for example, communities which heal and become healed in one and the same action.

CASE STUDIES IN SCARCITY AND SYNERGY

In this section we will consider three case studies in Western health care. Each examines the generation and distribution of health care resources within both a scarcity and synergy paradigm, demonstrating the interactions between the paradigms and the difficulties and opportunities for encouraging synergy in Western health care.

The Clinic and the Collective

In the first case study, we will consider the interactions a woman has with a medical clinic and a women's health collective. The clinic, operating primarily from within a scarcity paradigm, stresses the dissemination of *facts and information* about disease; the health collective, operating primarily within the synergy paradigm, stresses the support of patients' *knowledge*. With a growing concern for consumer awareness, we are witnessing an increased flow of data on disease that is packaged for dissemination to potential patients. Clinics begin this process even before they have definitive evidence that the potential patient has the disease he or she is being encouraged to learn about. But, facts about the disease are not automatic keys to empowerment. It is in the way patients make sense of the facts by viewing their sickness in a context that patients are empowered. When information or facts regarding disease are shared within a synergistic paradigm, illness can provide the opportunity for connectedness; it can bring people together to be empowered.

Anne, a woman in her early 20s had a consultation with her physician whom she had been seeing for several years; this visit was for what seemed to be a minor symptom: burning in the vaginal area.[3] After a brief examination, during which he noted a small blister in the affected area, he commented: "This could be herpes, you know." Anne explained that this was unlikely since she had been in a monogamous relationship for the past several years, and her spouse had no symptoms. She asked if the blister could be caused by a fingernail laceration that may have subsequently become filled with fluid as she had recently started taking baths. He considered this information irrelevant for the moment. Anne concluded that he was being "professional" by focusing on the possibility of an infectious disease. Hence, certain procedures had to be followed.

Anne was assigned to a nurse practitioner because her physician felt the nurse knew a good deal more about herpes symptomatology and diagnoses then he. The nurse described herpes to Anne in some detail, as the medical department believed that patients should be fully informed about the diseases for which they were being tested. Several cultures were taken and Anne was told the results would take several days.

In the meantime, Anne went through the clinic's education program. She was given a package of articles, photos, and a videotape of a lecture on herpes, which she felt gave overly dramatic yet ambiguous information. After the program, Anne asked the nurse several questions about her own symptoms as they did not resemble the photos and slides she had seen. She also wanted to know how to protect family, friends, and house guests from the infection, and about typical responses people had to the disease. The nurse's answers were vague and indirect, and Anne started to get frustrated.

Over the next few days, Anne kept calling the lab for her test results. She was assured that they would call her as soon as the tests were ready. Yet she received no phone calls about the results of the first two tests. Only when she finally insisted that she be given the results directly, rather than through her nurse practitioner, was she told that one of the tests was positive. The reason for the delay in letting her know was that her nurse had gone on vacation without letting Anne or the lab know.

The positive result was on a general test that indicated exposure to herpes but did not distinguish between oral and genital herpes. The second test, which was specifically for genital herpes, was negative. Since Anne already knew that oral herpes was not a matter for concern, she felt relieved and elated. Her nurse expressed annoyance at her elation, and said that the tests had to be repeated in two weeks in order for there to be "no doubt." She hoped Anne "would not be disappointed then," meaning that Anne would learn she in fact had genital herpes.

In the meantime Anne's blister had disappeared but the tension of waiting was beginning to distress her. She decided to call some members of her women's group for support. They referred her to a women's health collective in her town.

The women in the collective were less focused on *procedures* for sharing information about the disease; yet Anne found that the information available there was similar to what she had already learned at the medical clinic. But there was a difference in the way that information was handled—how it was given out and how she received it. In her conversations with women in the collective, Anne noticed that there was no single "expert" on the issues of health and healing; all were experts in their particular, sometimes unique, ways. Whenever she found herself wanting to focus on one woman's perspective, the group would guide her toward interactions with several others in the collective and encourage her to hear their views. For example, some women talked about herpes as an inconvenience, others treated it as a "problem that could be managed successfully"; some were pragmatic about it, others empathic and emotional.

Also, where Anne felt "isolated" and separated from herself and others at the clinic—"we were all looking *at* my disease"—she felt integrated and connected to others and part of a larger whole in the collective. As she put it, "I felt accepted for the way I was." Anne realized she did not have to wait for the lab results in order to become acceptable to the collective and, by extension, to the larger community. The stigma of disease was alleviated; she felt "intact, not flawed."

The women at the health collective seemed to have a very different relationship to the information and to Anne as the patient. Anne described them as being confident that she could manage the disease if she should have it: "They were not invested in my having herpes, or not having it. But yet they seemed to care about me. . . . They treated me as essentially healthy, even if I happened to have herpes."

Anne wondered why she felt differently about the nurse. She did not believe that the nurse "wanted me to be ill," but, she added, "the nurse did want something from me. She wanted to keep inundating me with information about herpes." In contrast, the collective focused more on enabling Anne:

> They cared more about giving me information that addressed my questions, like, how would herpes impact on my relationships? I felt isolated when I listened to the nurse. I felt handicapped, a threat to those I love. I had a contagious disease and felt I was to blame. The people at the collective

began with these issues. They knew where to begin. I don't
want information for its own sake. . . . They helped me pick
and choose the facts about herpes that answered *my* concerns,
such as, how would it effect my sexual relations with my
husband, what might his reactions be. . . . I felt comforted,
less alone.

Anne felt an issue of power with the nurse, where she as the patient
had the potential to give or take away a feeling of competence in the
nurse.

The final round of tests came back negative again. The nurse told
Anne "it doesn't mean a whole lot" because this was known to
occur in some cases where the patient did have herpes. She said
they would "have to act as if" Anne did not have herpes "until the
symptoms recur."

What implications can be drawn from this first case study about
synergistic healing in Western society? It might seem that the
contrast between the clinic and the health collective is overdrawn.
Unfortunately, the case is real. Women are confronted with clinics
like the one described more often than is commonly known (see
e.g., Boston Women's Health Book Collective, 1976; Ehrenreich &
English, 1978; Harrison, 1983). At the same time, the clinic is not
devoid of synergy, nor is the collective devoid of scarcity; the
contrast is based on a *relative* difference. The collective itself may
seem a "pale" example of synergistic community, especially when
compared to the drama of a !Kung healing dance, which is totally
integrated into and expressive of the culture. The collective is
synergistic primarily *in contrast* to the clinic. Existing without the
pervasive support of the culture at large, the collective illustrates
how synergy in the West often must build from a series of smaller,
more modest experiences.

The procedures for the testing of herpes are followed immaculately
at the clinic, but care for the person of the patient seems absent. The
physician does not seem to want to know how Anne must be feeling
and how she may be understanding what he is saying. He may believe
that concern detracts from efficiency in managing his patient load.
Empathy leads to a sense of liminality and vulnerability in the
provider as well as in the patient; a connection is forged, and the
sharing of care becomes more possible. But health providers often
believe such feelings are not essential to the health care process and
will at times attempt to curb them.

The clinic emphasizes treating the physical symptoms; it acts as if the patient's sense of well-being is not necessary for health. The clinic thus becomes an environment for disease management instead of health maintenance. Functioning within a scarcity paradigm, providers at the clinic act on the assumption that health is a scarce resource to which patients, i.e., "sick persons," aspire but often do not attain. If this assumption proves to be incorrect, providers at the clinic ironically experience themselves as diminished rather than enhanced. The women's health collective operates on the opposite assumption: if a client is healthy, or if she feels her needs can be addressed, then they are enhanced as a group. The collective emphasizes more the enabling of clients as its reason for existence, where the clinic believes more that the persistence of illness justifies its existence as a service.

There is no dearth of information available to Anne about the disease, its treatment, and its management. In fact, she is inundated with information. When she starts to question the impact of the possible herpes on *her own life,* the nurse cannot adequately respond. Yet, *only when* these questions are addressed at the women's collective does Anne feel more empowered.

This raises an important issue about information and consumer education. We have assumed that access to facts and multiple perspectives and the free flow of information is necessary to synergy (Katz, 1983/84); this may be a minimum requirement. It was in the *multiplicity* of approaches to herpes offered by the collective that Anne found support which, in a synergistic manner, was expanding and became renewable. She realized that there was no scarcity of responses to herpes which were valid and helpful—there were "many ways to have herpes." In combining these alternative responses, some of which were theoretically in conflict, she forged her own overall treatment-prevention response which was far greater than the sum of the individual responses and, accordingly, more helpful to her (see Katz & Rolde, 1981).

In a zero-sum view of empowerment, where scarcity implies that to the extent one person has information the other does not, the excessive giving of information may be a means to fend off a sense of powerlessness on the part of the caregiver. Within this scarcity paradigm, for the caregiver to receive information—for instance, by listening to the patient in order to learn more about the patient's needs—may be experienced as too disempowering a position for the caregiver to tolerate. It is the scarcity paradigm of the information "haves" and "have-nots," but with a twist: the imparting of information becomes an exercise in the pursuit of "power over" the other. If the information given is excessive, irrelevant, or distracting, the receiver will feel disempowered.

Though the *information* provided by the collective was in many instances similar to that provided by the clinic, the collective provided something else which was essential to healing: assisting Anne in her effort to turn random *information* into *personal knowledge* that related to her life and relationships. While lab reports and tests are key to diagnosis in modern medicine, they are not in themselves sufficient for healing to occur. A positive result on a test does not necessarily lead to a discontinuity in a client's sense of health; conversely, a negative result does not automatically lead to a feeling of health. Despite the fact the tests showed she did not have herpes, Anne was left with a feeling of ill health. Only through participating in the collective, as information was transformed into knowledge, did she feel healed. When information is shared in the context of synergy, access to information becomes helpful. Consumers do not need just information; they need to make meaning out of it and to fit it into their lives.

Anne says she feels "isolated," "rejected," and "to blame" for her symptoms. These feelings are not unusual in times of vulnerability and stress. They also point to the need for a perspective of self-in-community, especially in situations of illness. When Anne goes to the collective she feels less isolated; they do not require her to assume the role of patient so they can be the experts working on her needs. Rather, they stress a process of collaboration in addressing issues of concern so that a sense of empowerment is encouraged in all *who* participate. The process of collaboration then validates the existence of the health collective which leads to the continued existence of an empowering environment for the collective. This is synergy at work.

Is There Healing in Hospitals?

As in the case of the women's health collective, examples of synergistic community in Western health care tend to be set apart from the mainstream, often serving as a critique or a disturbing reminder of inadequacies in the system at large. Such communities are worthy of consideration because they can stimulate changes in that larger system as well as providing synergistic health care for their members.

Marie Balter's life story demonstrates the emergence of synergistic community within the walls of a state mental hospital (see Balter & Katz, 1986). Marie had been incarcerated in a state mental hospital for nearly twenty years, with only brief stays outside. Originally admitted at age 16 because of suicidal tendencies, she was officially diagnosed in her early 30s as schizophrenic. Marie was labelled a "hopeless case." Many in the hospital believed in that label, treating her as a "sick patient," and by such treatment withholding healing resources from her. Her care was reduced to medication, routine housekeeping assistance, and occasional and sporadic consultations with psychiatrists. Except for the medication, these healing resources were limited, and with the large hospital population, there were never enough resources to go around.

Though labelled "hopeless," Marie never fully lost her hope. Even when consumed by anxieties and hallucinations, she still kept alive an awareness of her condition and a motivation to get better. A few others at the hospital—several nurses, several volunteers and one of the psychiatrists—saw this inner life in Marie, and they too refused to accept the label of "hopeless." They offered help which went beyond the hospital routine, doing their jobs with care, and even love. They encouraged the hope they saw in Marie and expected her—though not fully—to be able to help herself.

At a point when she was perhaps the most disturbed and distressed—catatonic and severely depressed—the 36 year old Marie reached a painful conclusion:

> I began to be afraid of everything. I began to realize I had come to a point where I was so sick that I might not get well. Suddenly it would hit me: I was really crazy, I was in that world the nurses were always talking about.
>
> I remember saying to myself, "This is what I've come to. . . . I want to get out of it . . . but is it too late? Can I do it?"
>
> It got to the point where there was so much pain I had to make a decision whether to survive or not. I decided to fight back. I decided I wanted to get well. I decided I must get well or I might never leave that hospital.

With this realization, Marie took her first movements toward health in nearly a year. She began making her bed in order to regain a sense of normal touch in hands which had become numb. She played cards with the nurse who had been a long-time friend in order to engage in communication. She went to the hospital chapel and prayed: "Dear God, please help me . . . and if I get better I want to do everything I can to help other's who suffer like I do."

Now fueled by a renewed faith and an intense motivation to get better—both of which became healing resources which were expanding—Marie and others around her were more able to generate and regenerate helping situations and responses. A synergistic community formed—at different times and in different situations—which helped bring about her release from the hospital.

Marie remains out of the hospital, a productive and highly respected mental health worker—and it is now nearly twenty years since her release. Though the particular network of people which formed the hospital's healing environment for Marie no longer exists, specific persons in that network remain in contact with Marie and each other. Occasionally several persons gather with Marie, talking about the "good old times"—and the "bad times"—renewing the experience of a shared healing environment.

Through her professional work and personal character, Marie has been a beneficial influence on the local state hospital and mental health care throughout the state. As Marie says:

> Never write anyone off, no matter how hopeless they seem. You'll want to . . . but you never know. They took bets on me that I would return, and maybe they were right because I didn't behave that well, but look . . . I made it!

The lesson of hope entails a respect for the healing resources within each person. When encouraged, such self-generated resources can become renewable and can generate healing responses and eventually healing resources from others. Synergy then prevails.

The School as a Healing Environment

Synergy is said to exist in all communities. But a basic shift in perspective and understanding is needed to transform a community from one characterized by scarcity to one characterized by synergy. Marie Balter's story demonstrates one way such a shift can occur: by becoming a source and resource of hope for health rather than despair, she initiates this transformation. Karl, a young autistic child, demonstrates a similar pattern, but the shift occurs as a result of a more contrived intervention. Sometimes, the tenacity of the scarcity paradigm demands such an intervention if it is to yield to synergy.

Karl is 8 years old. From the age of 4, he has been clinically diagnosed as autistic.[4] A large boy, his movements have a jerky, unpredictable quality. His size accentuates the typical response others, especially his peers, have to him—he confuses them as he retreats from them in fear, and when he makes one of his infrequent gestures toward communication, he scares them away.

After having spent parts of his 5th and 6th year in various mental health settings, he entered first grade in public school when he was seven. His parents were hoping the school would become a helpful, healing environment for Karl. His mother put it this way: "We know he is really a lot like the other kids. If they could just treat him that way, we believe he can come out more and start to get better."

When Karl entered school, he was accompanied by a companion who assisted him in negotiating school tasks and acted as his interpreter and guide when others sought communication with him. Aside from his companion and his teacher, no one really attempted to help Karl; few attempted to communicate with him. He was ignored and excluded, considered an oddity, even an object of ridicule. He scared people and scared them away, largely through his own frightened responses. Also, Karl's companion, who acted as his gatekeeper, felt a need to "protect" him from this uncaring, even hostile, environment. As a result, what healing resources might have been available to Karl during his first grade experience were limited, as was his access to them. The year went by without major trauma but without any noticeable change in Karl's status.

During the summer, after reflecting on the completed school year, Karl's parents selected a different approach. They were committed to developing the school into a more responsive environment, one which would offer Karl care as well as concern. A family move necessitated a change in schools, and his parents took this opportunity to introduce a "new" Karl to the world.

They prepared a little booklet which introduced Karl to others at his new school. On the first page it said:

> Hello. My name is Karl. I want to be your friend. Sometimes you may think I act a little different, but that's because I don't feel well sometimes, and sometimes I'm scared. But I really want to be your friend. I hope we can get to know each other and play together.

The booklet went on to give specific suggestions on how best to interact with Karl so as to establish communication. For example, Karl offered this advice in it:

> A lot of times, I sit alone. Sometimes I want to be by myself. But I also want to play. If you want to play with me, its best not to take me by surprise, to come from behind me, or to come over too quickly, or come too close too quickly. That can scare me. Sometimes I may reach out to you and be a little rough. Please don't be scared, I'm just trying to say hello.

The booklet also discussed Karl's general psychological condition, placing the specific difficulties and challenges of communicating with him into context.

Written in large letters and in simple English, the booklet looked like an early grade reader. It included a friendly, smiling photo of Karl as well as a few photos of him at home and playing with peers. Children in Karl's grade commented upon how much they enjoyed reading it.

Karl's parents enlisted the support of the principal in disseminating the booklet and creating a context for its effective use. Meetings, in small groups, were held with all members of the school community, including students, teachers, custodial staff, and administrators. Discussion focused on how to make the entire school a healing environment, not just for Karl, but with Karl serving as an initial stimulus. An assumption was made explicit: in helping Karl, others could be helped and could learn to help each other. The booklet was offered as a *specific* guide to becoming helpful to one person and as a *general* model of how persons could become helpful to each other.

Karl's second grade experience was quite different. As well as there being no major traumas, Karl also showed an improved degree and ease of communication. The school community's commitment to help, aided by the practical suggestions in the booklet, multiplied the helping resources available to Karl. Karl became more a person to be helped rather than rejected or ignored, a person who wished to reach out rather than push away. The school context became one of potential communication rather than mutual fear. Everybody in the school was invited to become a source of help so that the community functioned more as a whole and had its potential for help exponentially increased. As Karl was presented as someone who wanted to connect with others ("I want to be your friend"), others were given the opportunity to be helpers and healers, which further encouraged Karl to present himself as someone wishing connection.

As others approached Karl with care and sensitivity, Karl responded with less fear, encouraging them even further. His peers set the tone; they displayed their sensitivity not in any dramatic "sensitive acts" but in just playing with Karl with a special concern for his interaction idiosyncrasies—and soon those idiosyncrasies became less important. Karl was not so easily frightened by abrupt movements. The process of communication fed upon itself and expanded. Helping Karl and seeing the success of those efforts empowered others as it empowered Karl; the helping cycle spread to other persons in the community—Karl modeled what was possible with others and the model was attempted many times. Karl's companion remained with him but now he had to protect Karl less and could care for him more. The companion was now letting people into Karl's world and letting Karl out into other's worlds. Many others now could offer the concern and care which the companion had before assumed almost singlehandedly.

Whereas Karl's first grade experience was characterized by the scarcity paradigm, limiting the healing resources available to himself *and* others, his second grade experience was characterized more by the synergy paradigm. By becoming himself an object *and* a source of helping, Karl helped his new school become more of a healing environment. As more members of the school community were able to help, the helping resources expanded. As Karl responded with his own communication, and the acts of helping Karl helped the helpers, helping resources at the school also became renewable. Karl was not cured in his second year at school. But the potential for his healing and the potential for the school to become a preventive environment was established.

SYNERGY IN WESTERN HEALING:
PRESENT STATUS, FUTURE CHALLENGE

Typically, synergistic healing communities in the West form in response to deficits in mainstream health care or in response to crisis; they occur within oppressed or disenfranchised groups, marginal to establishment health care systems, and offer an alternative or supplement to established procedures; and they exist within a larger non-synergistic environment which often devalues their worth and effectiveness. Synergy is never totally absent in a community if that community is to continue. But Western health care systems are characterized by a relative absence of synergy, reflecting the larger context of middle-class society.

The relative absence of synergy in Western health care and its occurrence primarily within disenfranchised communities do not constitute insurmountable barriers to the spread of synergy and its influence on mainstream systems. The areas in which synergy already occurs, such as support systems and indigenous healing systems, can be the *actual* foundation for its further development. Synergy can be worked with as a practical and viable response to the scarcity paradigm rather than as an instance of romantic, wishful thinking.

Support systems such as self-help groups are often paradigmatic synergistic communities within the Western health care system. Their mandated sharing of resources is usually buttressed by an egalitarian social structure (Katz & Bender, 1976). Alcoholics Anonymous is a classic example (Alcoholics Anonymous, 1955). Honest self-disclosure—telling one's story candidly—is a valued resource in the group; expertise in the group is synonymous with that honest sharing. Therefore, all members are potentially experts and have access to the valued resource. An egalitarian generation and distribution of valued resources prevails, enhanced by the anonymous nature of the group. Only with such honesty can one help oneself; only by helping oneself does one help others. One's story becomes a shared resource, stimulating group members to connect with one another and better understand their own experience. Support groups are often based on the sharing of an expanding and renewable healing resource.

Support groups also demonstrate the principles of synergy in another sense—they are often renewable and expanding in that they reproduce themselves and spawn offshoot groups and associated activities. For example, a group of Lupus Erythematosus (Lupus) patients gathered in an East Coast urban area in the late 1960s. Their intention was to help each other deal with a fundamental problem— they were not receiving good medical care, or even proper attention, from the medical establishment because physicians were generally misinformed about the disease. These patients, who were all women, were being told by their doctors that they had a primarily mental or emotional problem. But, though the understanding of Lupus was at that time still in its infancy, there was one local researcher-physician who understood more fully the physical basis and nature of the illness.

The original group, which offered psychological support and concrete advice on appropriate medical care as prescribed by the researcher-physician, decided to expand its purpose. Members initiated the formation of two other largely educational groups, one for relatives of Lupus patients, a second for interested physicians. The effects of the original group were felt, further stimulating the formation of a state Lupus organization, which exerted pressure on health policy issues, a national Lupus network, connecting the many state organizations which had developed on the model of the original state organization, and a foundation which raised money for research projects on Lupus. Some of the women from the original group, motivated by their earlier successes in the area of Lupus, also formed a coalition within the state with other citizens to lobby for improved health care for a wide range of illnesses and for specific protections for health consumers. And most important, the actual number of grass roots support groups of Lupus patients grew within the state and nationally and internationally. Like many self-help groups, it all started with one local group; as long as such groups continue to exist, the potential for renewable healing resources for Lupus patients continues.

Synergistic community is also characteristic of traditionally oriented or indigenous health systems, such as the healing ceremonies in Native American communities (e.g., Niehardt, 1972; Lame & Erdoes, 1972) and Espiritismo and Santeria in the Latino community (e.g., Comas-Diaz, 1981; Delgado, 1978). Healing ceremonies among the Lakota Sioux on the Rosebud and Pine Ridge Reservations, and the traditional spiritual knowledge out of which the ceremonies grow, are resources meant to be shared and renewed. Though preserved and developed primarily by the elders and others who have cultural wisdom such as medicine people, traditional knowledge is a community resource. It is meant to be shared throughout the community, provided there is a respectful attitude toward receiving it.

Passed on from generation to generation among the Lakota, this traditional spiritual knowledge becomes renewable, and renews the community (Brown, 1953; Niehardt, 1972). For example, on his "vision quest," a Lakota learns about himself, his culture, and his place in his community; during the vision quest, he prays so that his people will not suffer. The community is the prime recipient of knowledge gained during this sacred ceremony and the healing from it. As one returns from the hill where the vision quest was made, one is brought back into the community; the stories brought back from the vision quest enlarge the community's understanding of itself (Lame Deer & Erdoes, 1972). Fed by the performances of the ceremonies like the vision quest, the community is better able to support subsequent ceremonies, regenerating their occurrence.

Indigenous health systems are considered marginal by mainstream health care professionals; this is the case even when they are effective with clients. But this evaluation seems derived largely from the fact that these indigenous systems exist within communities which are usually disempowered and oppressed. Being different from mainstream services and *practiced within disempowered communities*, it is thought that these indigenous systems can be dismissed. But rather than being marginal, these indigenous systems are essential; rather than being dismissed, we must turn to them and learn from them because they offer health care within a synergistic paradigm which meets clients' needs.

A third situation in which synergistic community is more likely to exist in present Western health care systems is during times of crisis. Synergistic communities frequently arise in response to moments of crisis, whether it be from some external threat, high intensity task commitment, or an emergency internal to group functioning. The Outward Bound Schools have attempted to provide such an environment with their program of challenge education (Katz & Kolb, 1972). A major problem with Outward Bound is the transitory nature of the synergy experienced and the restricted transfer of that experience to situations outside of Outward Bound— a problem typical with intense, crisis-oriented groups such as task forces working on a deadline.

The blizzard of 1978 in the Northeast provided an example of how synergy can not only occur as a response to a crisis but can also be built into an ongoing health system. Throughout the affected area, people were brought together to work on common problems. With public transportation disrupted and most work places closed, urban neighborhoods became neighborly as people worked to dig out their cars and walkways, the healthy and capable offering to help those neighbors who, because of age, infirmity, or family situation, could not cope with the storm. People spent time in the middle of the street—which, closed to vehicular traffic, now served as a village common—exchanging stories about the storm's effects. One person expressed a feeling which was frequently heard: "This storm is really something! I never thought the storm could bring such a nice feeling to the neighborhood. It just shows that when we work together, we can accomplish quite a bit."

In an urban neighborhood in Boston, this common response to the crisis of the storm was translated into an enduring structure. This neighborhood, with a predominantly working-class Irish-American composition, had difficulty in receiving quality care from and equitable access to the local community health center, which had a university connection and orientation. There was a conflict between the center and its immediate neighborhood which resulted in minimal use of the center.

As a continuation of discussions in the street during the storm, a group of neighborhood people began meeting informally. They tried to direct their experiences during the storm of "functioning beyond the self" toward improving the health center. They developed concrete plans to open the center to more community input and bring it more into the mainstream of community life. New and culturally sensitive services were proposed and combinations of alternative and existing services were suggested. As the center put these plans into action, not only was the center utilized more and the quality of service improved, but also the center began serving as an enduring structure to bring a sense of synergy to the neighborhood—a reciprocating effect was established.

How might synergy be more systematically encouraged—both within these settings where it already occurs and in other settings? Given the pervasive influence of the larger social context of Western culture with its emphasis on scarcity, this is partly a question of social policy.

Of primary importance is a shift away from the scarcity paradigm toward the synergy paradigm. At present, scarcity-based models dominate the planning of change and, to the extent that plans guide actual interventions, the process of change itself (e.g., Rappaport, 1985). Social action theorists within the scarcity paradigm are concerned with the more equitable redistribution of *limited* resources, cutting up the *limited* pie in a more equitable manner. Berger (1976), for example, describes the classic dilemma in such scarcity-based models when he talks about the sacrifices necessary in any process of change, because change always involves "losers" when there are "winners."

A model of change based on the synergy paradigm does not employ the image of a limited or fixed pie because the valued resources are seen as renewable and expanding. When change is introduced all involved can be "winners." Processes of change which release such expanding and renewable resources are documented by Seth (1986) and Reichmann (1985). For example, family planning efforts in rural India are more effective and more humane when women are involved in self-organized discussions about fertility options rather than, as in the usual manner, merely being told about these options or convinced to use one of them (Seth, 1986). The women become sources as well as recipients of knowledge about fertility options. When women are thus empowered, knowledge about fertility is rapidly and effectively passed on from woman to woman.

A second area of importance in encouraging synergy is the nature of the intervention strategy employed, including the nature of the change agent. One way to encourage synergy is through intentional and purposive change. The environment can be intentionally restructured to evoke synergy rather than scarcity as in the cases of Dr. Fendor, Marie, and Karl.

More specifically, the environment can be intentionally restructured so that differing, sometimes conflicting, health services are brought together in a context in which they work in harmony to produce a larger, more synergistic whole (Katz & Rolde, 1981); such an intervention is illustrated earlier in the case of the women's health collective.

Rappaport's (1981) call for divergent instead of convergent thinking and planning in community psychology offers another example of this intentional strategy. Convergent thinking tends to limit options and reinforce old planning strategies, even though they may be ineffective. With divergent thinking, new *and* differing plans emerge, increasing the likelihood that more effective planning can be constructed from some combinations of diverse ideas.

But synergy, as Fuller (1969) states, is "already there"; it represents the natural, intrinsic condition of the universe. Therefore, one is also led to support a second concept of intervention to encourage synergy, what might be called a "non-interventionist" or releasing strategy. If we assume that communities and individuals have significant self-healing capacities (e.g., Davis, 1976), then the task of the change agent is to facilitate the release of those capacities or, more bluntly, not to interfere with natural healing resources. In fact, the term "change agent" becomes somewhat inappropriate, particularly if it implies a person or organization possessing professional expertise which must be activated if change is to occur. In the non-interventionist strategy, expertise becomes a shared resource, originating in and available to all members of the community. The community becomes its own change agent, removing the separation between the changed and changer and introducing a powerful concept of prevention. Those with special skills in "intervention" or "consultation" can still be valuable, but their skill is offered within the context of the community, as a resource of the community.

This model of the change agent as a non-interventionist can be a powerful political force, moving health care toward a synergistic paradigm. The collaborative nature of this approach transforms an intervention into a participatory exchange and undercuts the persistent power differentials necessary for the scarcity paradigm. But this model of the change agent also produces difficulties in the training of helpers and others concerned with social change; in the place of the present exclusive training emphasis on competence, there would have to be a complementary emphasis on vulnerability.

A third area of importance in encouraging synergy in Western health care focuses on the education of helpers and caregivers. The training model emphasizes that the caregiver establish a professional distance from clients and develop a sense of competence which often devolves into a sense of omnipotence (e.g., Cheever, 1985; Light, 1980). Clients or patients, therefore, become "persons who need to be helped," and since they do not possess expert knowledge about their problem, their input into treatment is of minimal value. In contrast, synergy in health care would be encouraged if caregivers were educated within a synergistic paradigm (Cheever, 1985; Seyal, 1986; Simonis, 1985). With this synergistically-oriented training, health providers are taught to appreciate their own vulnerability and to understand how the maintenance of health is a shared responsibility between themselves, clients, and communities (Katz, 1981, 1986; Light, 1980). The provider can then participate with the client in generating a combination of healing resources—from the provider, the client, the community—which could be larger than the sum of the parts (Katz & Rolde, 1981).

"Education as transformation" (Katz, 1981)—a model of traditional healer education—is one way in which such vulnerability and shared responsibility can be taught (Hampton, 1986; Nunez-Molina, 1985). "Education as transformation" stresses that character must precede and serve as the context for technical knowledge, and that the healer must be trained to serve the community. At the University of Alaska/Fairbanks, we are developing a community psychology program guided by this transformational model. The dilemma is to integrate a model of education based on traditional principles of oral cultures into the university, an institution committed to "modernity" and "essayist literacy." But there is evidence that education as transformation is viable within the university (see, e.g., Simonis's [1985] research on the university education of counselors and Cheever's [1984] review of the education of community mental health workers).

Given the essential requirement that resources be shared on a global scale if the human community is to survive, the sharing of health resources becomes a necessity. Otherwise, the health care system is not truly healing. Synergy, with its release of renewable and expanding resources, is a future necessity. Synergistic community, which provides the process and structure within which these renewable and expanding resources are accessed equitably by all members, can introduce a low-cost, pervasive mode of health care, which reestablishes a sense of human community.

But the scarcity, not the synergy, paradigm dominates mainstream Western approaches to healing. Health care has become a scarce resource; people must compete for access to it—and the result is inequitable access. Mainstream approaches reflect the values of the culture within which they function; therefore, if we wish to encourage synergy in Western healing, we must consider larger cultural and political issues. Present socio-political structures do not seem adequate for meeting those health needs which require shared resources.

The introduction of synergistic community could help us move away from the present Western emphasis on competition for scarce, expert-generated treatment techniques toward an emphasis on sharing renewable, community-generated prevention patterns. To insure that synergy releases resources which are healing, we have to guard against situations where the very existence of synergy is used by the larger society as an avenue of oppression, and where synergy is a mask for exploitation within and between groups.

Rappaport (1978) provides another perspective on the need for synergy. He suggests that over the course of human evolution, rituals in which we overcome our separateness and experience a transpersonal bonding have been necessary for the survival of the species. These rituals enable us to accomplish those communal tasks which guarantee the continuity of the human community. The individualism and consequent fragmentation of these communal efforts in contemporary Euro-American industrialized society is well-documented (e.g., Berger, Berger & Kellner, 1973). Synergistic community offers an alternative to this fragmentation, stressing a transpersonal bonding within a supportive socio-cultural context.

NOTES

1. Dr. Fendor is a pseudonym. The case study is based on data collected in 1985 as part of an informal study of Freirean approaches to health and education.
2. Terms such as the "West" and "Western" can be confusing. We are using these terms to refer to contemporary, mainstream Euro-American culture, which dominates western Europe and North America, but which is expressed in some form in most parts of the world. These terms, therefore, refer to a particular cultural context rather than a specific geographic location.
3. Anne is a pseudonym. The case study is based on data collected in 1982 to provide material on issues of synergy and health care.
4. Karl is a pseudonym. The case study is based on data collected in the early 1980s during a school consultation.

REFERENCES

Alcoholics Anonymous. (1955). *Alcoholics anonymous*. New York: Alcoholics Anonymous World Services.

Balter, M. & Katz, R. (1986). *Sing no sad songs*. Unpublished manuscript, Harvard University, Cambridge.

Berger, P. (1976). *Pyramids of sacrifice: Political ethics and social change*. Garden City, NY: Doubleday Anchor Books.

Berger, P., Berger, B. & Kellner, H. (1973). *The homeless mind: Modernization and consciousness*. New York: Random House.

Brint, S. (1981). Knowledge and work, knowledge and power: The promise and problems of "new class" theories. *Harvard Educational Review, 51* (4), 587-596.

Brown, J. E. (1953). *The sacred pipe: Black Elk's account of the seven rites of the Oglala Sioux*. Norman, OK: University of Oklahoma.

Boston Women's Health Book Collective. (1976). *Our bodies, our selves*. New York: Simon & Schuster.

Cheever, O. (1984). *The education of community psychiatrists: A search for transcultural community-based models*. Qualifying paper, Harvard Graduate School of Education, Cambridge.

Comas-Diaz, L. (1981). Puerto Rican Espiritismo and psychotherapy. *American Journal of Orthopsychiatry, 51*(4).

Davies, M. (1976). Systems theory and social work. In J. Beishon & G. Peters (eds.), *Systems behavior*. New York: Harper & Row.

Delgado, M. (1978). Folk medicine in the Puerto Rican culture. *International Journal of Social Work, 21*, 45-54.

Ehrenreich, B. & English, D. (1978). *For her own good: 150 years of the experts advice to women*. Garden City, NY: Anchor Press.

Freire, P. (1968). *Pedagogy of the oppressed*. New York: Seabury Press.

Fuller, B. (1963). *Ideas and integrities*. New York: Macmillan.

Goffman, E. (1961). *Asylums*. New York: Anchor.

Hampton, E. (1986). *Toward an Indian model of education*. Doctoral thesis, Harvard Graduate School of Education, Cambridge.

Harrison, M. (1983). *A woman in residence*. New York: Penguin Books.

Harron, F., Burnside, J. & Beauchamp, T. (1983). *Health and human values: A guide to making your own decisions*. New Haven: Yale University Press.

James, W. (1963). *The varieties of religious experiences*. New York: Modern Library.

Katz, A. & Bender, E. (eds.) (1976). *The strength in us: Self-help groups in the modern world*. New York: Franklin Watts.

Katz, R. (1981). Education as transformation: Becoming a healer among the !Kung and Fijians. *Harvard Educational Review, 51*(1), 57-78.

Katz, R. (1982). *Boiling energy: Community healing among the Kalahari !Kung*. Cambridge, MA: Harvard University Press.

Katz, R. (1983/84). Empowerment and synergy: Towards expanding community healing resources. *Prevention in Human Services, 3*(2/3), 201-225.

Katz, R. & Kilner, L. (in press). The straight path: A Fijian perspective on development. In C. Super & S. Harkness (eds.), *Studies in comparative human development*. New York: Academic Press.

Katz, R. & Kolb, D. (1972). Challenge to grow: The Outward Bound approach. In D. Purpel & M. Belanger (eds.), *Curriculum and the cultural revolution*. Berkeley: McCutchan Press.

Katz, R. & Nunez-Molina, M. (1986). Researching "realities": A method for understanding cultural diversity. *The Community Psychologist, 19*(2).

Katz, R. & Rolde, E. (1981). Community alternatives to psychotherapy. *Psychotherapy: Theory, Research and Practice, 18*(3), 365-374.

Lame Deer (John Fire) & Erdoes, R. (1972). *Lame Deer, seeker of visions: The life of a Sioux medicine man*. New York: Simon & Schuster.

Lee, R. (1979). *The !Kung San: Men, women and work in a foraging society*. Cambridge, England: Cambridge University Press.

Lee, R. & DeVore, I. (eds.) (1968). *Man the hunter*. Chicago: Aldine.

Marshall, L. (1969). The medicine dance of the !Kung Bushmen. *Africa, 39*.

Marshall, L. (1976). *The !Kung of Nyae Nyae*. Cambridge, MA: Harvard University Press.

Maslow, A. & Honigmann, J. (1970). Ruth Benedict's notes on synergy. *American Anthropologist, 72*.

Niehardt, J. (1972). *Black Elk speaks*. New York: Pocket Books.

Nunez-Molina, M. (1985). *The education of the healer in Puerto Rican Espiritismo*. Qualifying paper, Harvard Graduate School of Education, Cambridge.

Polanyi, M. (1964). *Personal knowledge: Towards a post-critical philosophy*. New York: Harper & Row.

Rappaport, J. (1981). In praise of paradox: A social policy of empowerment over prevention. *American Journal of Community Psychology, 9*(1).

Rappaport, J. (1985). The power of empowerment language. *Social Policy*, Fall.

Rappaport, R. (1978). Adaptation and the structure of rituals. In N. Blurton-Jones & V. Reynolds (eds.), *Human Behavior and adaptation*. New York: Halstead Press.

Reichmann, R. (1985). *"Consciencia" and development: Tricicleros' grassroots labor organization in the Dominican Republic.* Thesis, Harvard Graduate School of Education, Cambridge.

Sarason, S. (1977). *The psychological sense of community: Prospects for a community psychology.* San Francisco: Jossey-Bass.

Seth, N. (1986). *"Baira ni vato" (women's talk): A context for exploring fertility options.* Doctoral thesis, Harvard Graduate School of Education, Cambridge.

Seyal, F. (1986). *Fountain House: A non-traditional psychiatric treatment program for chronic schizophrenics.* Qualifying paper, Harvard Graduate School of Education, Cambridge.

Simonis, J. (1985). Synergy and the education of healers: A new community psychology approach to counselor training. Doctoral thesis, Harvard Graduate School of Education, Cambridge.

Turner, V. (1969). *The ritual process.* Chicago: Aldine.

W.H.O. (1976). *Alma-Ata conference and declaration on primary health care.* New York: World Health Organization.